Marx Joyce
Abbott Hardy Montaigne Machiavelli Chesterton Cooper Emerson Austen
Defoe Melville Haggard Hugo
Christie Carroll Eliot Grimm
Stoker Molière
Wilde Maupassant Byron
Engels Schiller
Garnett Einstein Fitzgerald Smith
Goethe Hawthorne Kafka
Cotton Dostoyevsky Hall
Baum Kipling Doyle Willis
Leslie Dumas Henry Nietzsche
Flaubert Turgenev Balzac
Stockton Vatsyayana Crane
Burroughs Whitman
Verne
Curtis Tocqueville Gogol Vinci
Homer Widger Tolstoy Busch
Darwin Thoreau
Potter Freud Zola Twain Plato Scott
Lawrence
Kant Jowett Stevenson Dickens
Andersen Burton Hesse Harte
London Descartes Cervantes
Poe Aristotle Wells Voltaire
Hale James Hastings
Cooke
Bunner Shakespeare
Richter Chekhov Chambers Irving
da Shaw Wodehouse Benedict
Doré Swift Dante Alcott
Pushkin
Newton

tredition®

tredition was established in 2006 by Sandra Latusseck and Soenke Schulz. Based in Hamburg, Germany, tredition offers publishing solutions to authors and publishing houses, combined with worldwide distribution of printed and digital book content. tredition is uniquely positioned to enable authors and publishing houses to create books on their own terms and without conventional manufacturing risks.

For more information please visit: www.tredition.com

TREDITION CLASSICS

This book is part of the TREDITION CLASSICS series. The creators of this series are united by passion for literature and driven by the intention of making all public domain books available in printed format again - worldwide. Most TREDITION CLASSICS titles have been out of print and off the bookstore shelves for decades. At tredition we believe that a great book never goes out of style and that its value is eternal. Several mostly non-profit literature projects provide content to tredition. To support their good work, tredition donates a portion of the proceeds from each sold copy. As a reader of a TREDITION CLASSICS book, you support our mission to save many of the amazing works of world literature from oblivion. See all available books at www.tredition.com.

Project Gutenberg

The content for this book has been graciously provided by Project Gutenberg. Project Gutenberg is a non-profit organization founded by Michael Hart in 1971 at the University of Illinois. The mission of Project Gutenberg is simple: To encourage the creation and distribution of eBooks. Project Gutenberg is the first and largest collection of public domain eBooks.

Essentials of Diseases of the Skin Including the Syphilodermata Arranged in the Form of Questions and Answers Prepared Especially for Students of Medicine

Henry Weightman Stelwagon

Imprint

This book is part of TREDITION CLASSICS

Author: Henry Weightman Stelwagon
Cover design: Buchgut, Berlin – Germany

Publisher: tredition GmbH, Hamburg - Germany
ISBN: 978-3-8472-2581-2

www.tredition.com
www.tredition.de

The intention of the TREDITION CLASSICS series is to make world literature in the public domain available in printed format. Literary enthusiasts and organizations, such as Project Gutenberg, worldwide have scanned and digitally edited the original texts. tredition has subsequently formatted and redesigned the content into a modern reading layout. Therefore, we cannot guarantee the exact reproduction of the original format of a particular historic edition. Please also note that no modifications have been made to the spelling, therefore it may differ from the orthography used today.

DORLAND'S

AMERICAN ILLUSTRATED

MEDICAL DICTIONARY

For Students and Practitioners

A New and Complete Dictionary of the terms used in Medicine, Surgery, Dentistry, Pharmacy, Chemistry, and kindred branches; together with new and elaborate Tables of Arteries, Muscles, Nerves, Veins, etc.; of Bacilli, Bacteria, Micrococci, etc.; Eponymic Tables of Diseases, Operations, Signs and Symptoms, Stains, Tests, Methods of Treatment, etc. By W.A.N. Dorland, M.D., Editor of the American Pocket Medical Dictionary. Large octavo, nearly 800 pages, bound in full flexible leather. Price, $4.50 net; with thumb index, $5.00 net.

JUST ISSUED—NEW (4) REVISED EDITION--2000 NEW WORDS

It contains a maximum amount of matter in a minimum space and at the lowest possible cost.

This book contains **double the material in the ordinary students' dictionary**, and yet, by the use of a clear, condensed type and thin paper of the finest quality, is only 1-3/4 inches in thickness. It is bound in full flexible leather, and is just the kind of a book that a man will want to keep on his desk for constant reference. The book makes a special feature of **the newer words**, and defines hundreds of important terms not to be found in any other dictionary. It is especially **full in the matter of tables**, containing more than a hundred of great practical value, including new tables of Tests, Stains and Staining Methods. A new feature is the inclusion of numerous handsome illustrations, many of them in colors, drawn and engraved specially for this book.

"I must acknowledge my astonishment at seeing how much he has condensed within relatively small space. I find nothing to criticise, very much to commend, and was interested in finding some of the new words which are not in other recent dictionaries."—Roswell Park, *Professor of Principles and Practice of Surgery and Clinical Surgery, University of Buffalo.*

"Dr. Dorland's Dictionary is admirable. It is so well gotten up and of such convenient size. No errors have been found in my use of it."—Howard A. Kelly, *Professor of Gynecology, Johns Hopkins University, Baltimore.*

W. B. SAUNDERS COMPANY, 925 Walnut St., Phila.

London: 9, Henrietta Street, Covent Garden

Fifth Edition, Just Ready **With Complete Vocabulary**

THE

AMERICAN POCKET

MEDICAL DICTIONARY

EDITED BY

W.A. NEWMAN DORLAND, A.M., M.D.,

Assistant Demonstrator of Obstetrics, University of Pennsylvania.

HUNDREDS OF NEW TERMS

Bound in Full Leather, Limp, with Gold Edges. Price, $1.00 net; with Patent Thumb Index, $1.25 net.

The book is an **absolutely new one**. It is not a revision of any old work, but it has been written entirely anew and is constructed on lines that experience has shown to be the most practical for a work of this kind. It aims to be **complete**, and to that end contains practically all the terms of modern medicine. This makes an unusually large vocabulary. Besides the ordinary dictionary terms the book contains a wealth of **anatomical and other tables**. This matter is of particular value to students for memorizing in preparation for examination.

"I am struck at once with admiration at the compact size and attractive exterior. I can recommend it to our students without reserve." —James W. Holland, M.D., *of Jefferson Medical College*.

"This is a handy pocket dictionary, which is so full and complete that it puts to shame some of the more pretentious volumes." —*Journal of the American Medical Association*.

"We have consulted it for the meaning of many new and rare terms, and have not met with a disappointment. The definitions are exquisitely clear and concise. We have never found so much information in so small a space." —*Dublin Journal of Medical Science*.

"This is a handy little volume that, upon examination, seems fairly to fulfil the promise of its title, and to contain a vast amount of information in a very small space.... It is somewhat surprising that it contains so many of the rarer terms used in medicine." —*Bulletin Johns Hopkins Hospital*, Baltimore.

ESSENTIALS

OF

DISEASES OF THE SKIN.

Since the issue of the first volume of the Saunders Question-Compends,

OVER 290,000 COPIES

of these unrivalled publications have been sold. This enormous sale is indisputable evidence of the value of these self-helps to students and physicians.

SAUNDERS' QUESTION-COMPENDS. No. 11.

ESSENTIALS

OF

DISEASES OF THE SKIN

INCLUDING THE

SYPHILODERMATA

ARRANGED IN THE FORM OF

QUESTIONS AND ANSWERS

PREPARED ESPECIALLY FOR

STUDENTS OF MEDICINE

BY

HENRY W. STELWAGON, M.D., PH.D.

Professor of Dermatology in the Jefferson Medical College, Philadelphia; Dermatologist to the Howard and Philadelphia Hospitals, etc.

SEVENTH EDITION, THOROUGHLY REVISED

ILLUSTRATED

PHILADELPHIA AND LONDON

W. B. SAUNDERS COMPANY

1909

Set up, electrotyped, printed, 1890. Reprinted July, 1891.
Revised, reprinted, June, 1894. Reprinted March, 1897.
Revised, reprinted, August, 1899. Reprinted September,
1901, May, 1902, September, 1903. Revised, reprinted
January, 1905. Reprinted March,
1906. Revised, reprinted
March, 1909.

PRINTED IN AMERICA
PRESS OF
W. B. SAUNDERS COMPANY
PHILADELPHIA

PREFACE TO SEVENTH EDITION.

In the present—seventh—edition the subject matter, especially as regards the practical part, has been gone over carefully and the necessary corrections and additions made. Nineteen new illustrations have been added, a few of the old ones being eliminated. It is hoped that the continued demand for this compend means a widening interest in the study of diseases of the skin, sufficiently keen as to lead to the desire for a still greater knowledge.

H.W.S.

PREFACE TO FIRST EDITION.

Much of the present volume is, in a measure, the outcome of a thorough revision, remodelling and simplification of the various articles contributed by the author to Pepper's System of Medicine, Buck's Reference Handbook of the Medical Sciences, and Keating's Cyclopædia of the Diseases of Children. Moreover, in the endeavor to present the subject as tersely and briefly as compatible with clear understanding, the several standard treatises on diseases of the skin by Tilbury Fox, Duhring, Hyde, Robinson, Anderson, and Crocker, have been freely consulted, that of the last-named author suggesting the pictorial presentation of the "Anatomy of the Skin." The space allotted to each disease has been based upon relative importance. As to treatment, the best and approved methods only—those which are founded upon the aggregate experience of dermatologists—are referred to.

For general information a statistical table from the Transactions of the American Dermatological Association is appended.

H.W.S.

DISEASES OF THE SKIN.

ANATOMY OF THE SKINFig. 1.

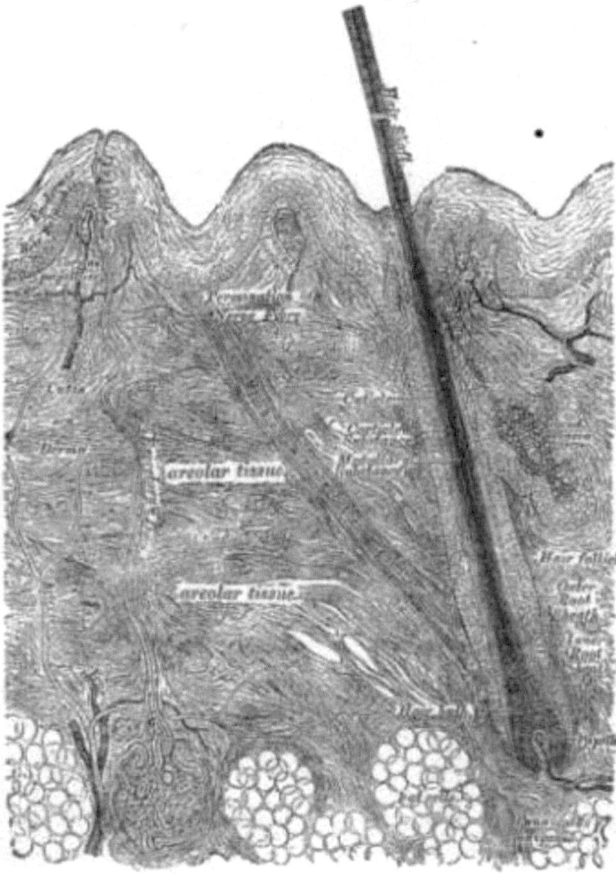

Vertical section of the skin—Diagrammatic. (*After Heitsmann.*)

The Epidermis.

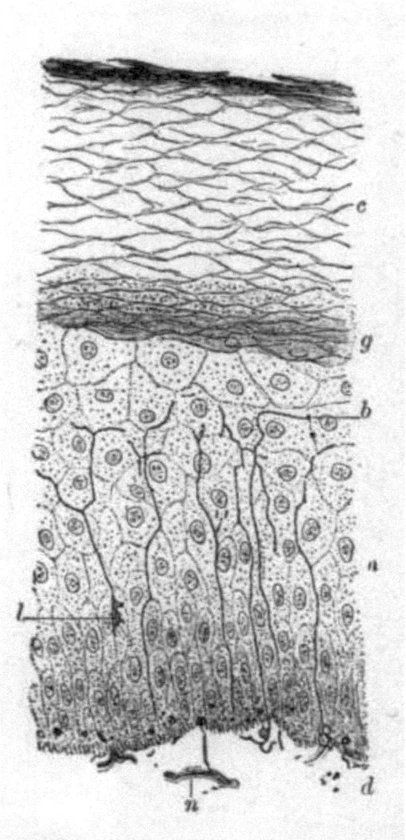

Fig. 2.

c, corneous (horny) layer; *g*, granular layer; *m*, mucous layer (rete Malpighii).
The stratum lucidum is the layer just above the granular layer.
Nerve terminations—*n*, afferent nerve; *b*, terminal nerve bulbs; *l*, cell of Langerhans.

(*After Ranvier.*)

The Blood-vessels.

Fig. 3.

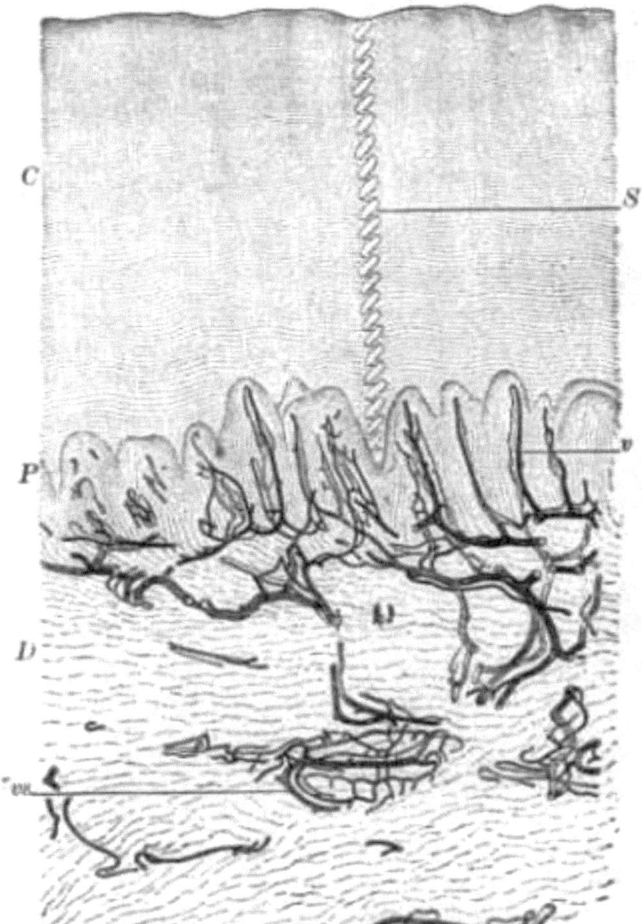

C, epidermis; *D*, corium; *P*, papillæ; *S*, sweat-gland duct.
v, arterial and venous capillaries (superficial, or papillary plexus) of the papillæ.
Deep plexus is partly shown at lower margin of the diagram; *vs*—an intermediate
plexus, an outgrowth from the deep plexus, supplying sweat-glands, and
giving a loop to hair papilla.

(*After Ranvier*).

[Pg 20]

The Nervous and Vascular Papillæ.

Fig. 4.

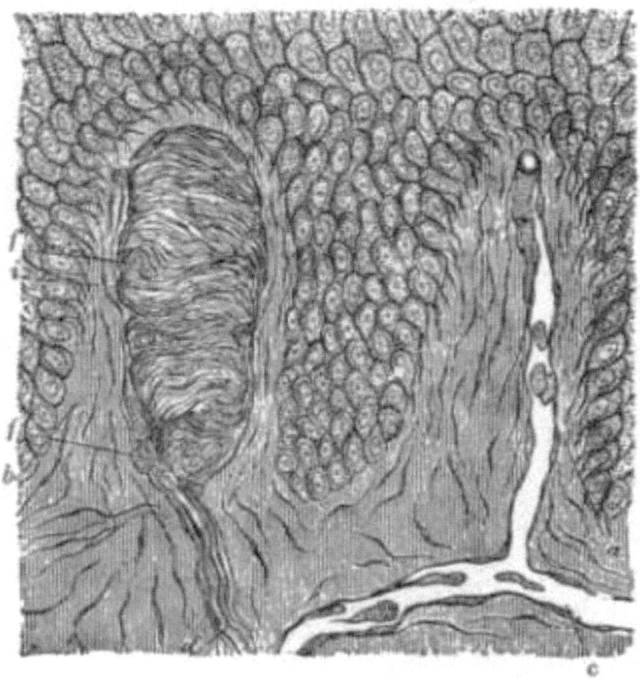

a, a vascular papilla; *b*, a nervous papilla; *c*, a blood-vessel; *d*, a nerve fibre;
e, a tactile corpuscle.

(*After Biesiadecki.*)

[Pg 21]

The Hair and Hair-Follicle.

Fig. 5.

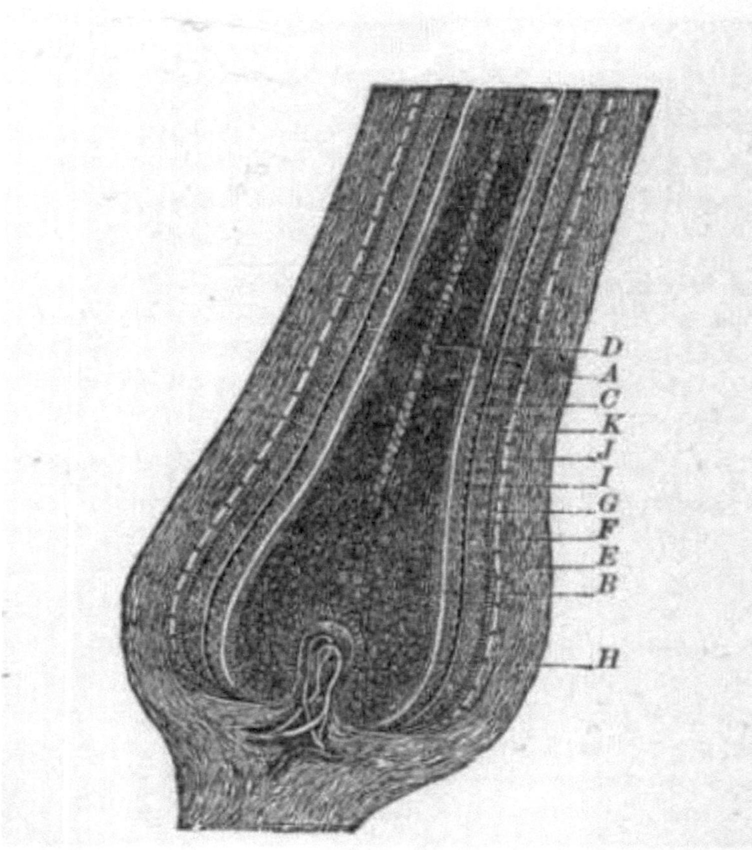

A, shaft of the hair; *B*, root of the hair; *C*, cuticle of the hair; *D*, medullary substance of the hair.

E, external layer of the hair-follicle; *F*, middle layer of the hair-follicle; *G*, internal layer of the hair-follicle; *H*, papilla of the hair; *I*, external root-sheath; *J*, outer layer of the internal root-sheath; *K*, internal layer of the internal root-sheath.

(*After Duhring.*)

[Pg 22]

SYMPTOMATOLOGY.

The symptoms of cutaneous disease may be objective, subjective or both; and in some diseases, also, there may be systemic disturbance.

What do you mean by objective symptoms?

Those symptoms visible to the eye or touch.

What do you understand by subjective symptoms?

Those which relate to sensation, such as itching, tingling, burning, pain, tenderness, heat, anæsthesia, and hyperæsthesia.

What do you mean by systemic symptoms?

Those general symptoms, slight or profound, which are sometimes associated, primarily or secondarily, with the cutaneous disease, as, for example, the systemic disturbance in leprosy, pemphigus, and purpura hemorrhagica.

Into what two classes of lesions are the objective symptoms commonly divided?

Primary (or elementary), and

Secondary (or consecutive).

Primary Lesions.

What are primary lesions?

Those objective lesions with which cutaneous diseases begin. They may continue as such or may undergo modification, passing into the secondary or consecutive lesions.

Enumerate the primary lesions.

Macules, papules, tubercles, wheals, tumors, vesicles, blebs and pustules.

What are macules (maculæ)?

Variously-sized, shaped and tinted spots and discolorations, without elevation or depression; as, for example, freckles, spots of purpura, macules of cutaneous syphilis. [Pg 23]

What are papules (papulæ)?

Small, circumscribed, solid elevations, rarely exceeding the size of a split-pea, and usually superficially seated; as, for example, the papules of eczema, of acne, and of cutaneous syphilis.

What are tubercles (tubercula)?

Circumscribed, solid elevations, commonly pea-sized and usually deep-seated; as, for example, the tubercles of syphilis, of leprosy, and of lupus.

What are wheals (pomphi)?

Variously-sized and shaped, whitish, pinkish or reddish elevations, of an evanescent character; as, for example, the lesions of urticaria, the lesions produced by the bite of a mosquito or by the sting of a nettle.

What are tumors (tumores)?

Soft or firm elevations, usually large and prominent, and having their seat in the corium and subcutaneous tissue; as, for example, sebaceous tumors, gummata, and the lesions of fibroma.

What are vesicles (vesiculæ)?

Pin-head to pea-sized, circumscribed epidermal elevations, containing serous fluid; as, for example, the so-called fever-blisters, the lesions of herpes zoster, and of vesicular eczema.

What are blebs (bullæ)?

Rounded or irregularly-shaped, pea to egg-sized epidermic elevations, with fluid contents; in short, they are essentially the same as vesicles and pustules except as to size; as, for example, the blebs of pemphigus, rhus poisoning, and syphilis.

What are pustules (pustulæ)?

Circumscribed epidermic elevations containing pus; as, for example, the pustules of acne, of impetigo, and of sycosis.

Secondary Lesions.

What are secondary lesions?

Those lesions resulting from accidental or natural change, modification or termination of the primary lesions. [Pg 24]

Enumerate the secondary lesions.

Scales, crusts, excoriations, fissures, ulcers, scars and stains.

What are scales (squamæ)?

Dry, laminated, epidermal exfoliations; as, for example, the scales of psoriasis, ichthyosis, and eczema.

What are crusts (crustæ)?

Dried effete masses of exudation; as, for example, the crusts of impetigo, of eczema, and of the pustular and ulcerating syphilodermata.

What are excoriations (excoriationes)?

Superficial, usually epidermal, linear or punctate loss of tissue; as, for example, ordinary scratch-marks.

What are fissures (rhagades)?

Linear cracks or wounds, involving the epidermis, or epidermis and corium; as, for example, the cracks which often occur in eczema when seated about the joints, the cracks of chapped lips and hands.

What are ulcers (ulcera)?

Rounded or irregularly-shaped and sized loss of skin and subcutaneous tissue resulting from disease; as, for example, the ulcers of syphilis and of cancer.

What are scars (cicatrices)?

Connective-tissue new formations replacing loss of substance.

What are stains?

Discolorations left by cutaneous disease, which stains may be transitory or permanent.

Distribution and Configuration.

What do you mean by a patch of eruption?

A single group or aggregation of lesions or an area of disease.

When is an eruption said to be limited or localized?

When it is confined to one part or region. [Pg 25]

When is an eruption said to be general or generalized?

When it is scattered, uniformly or irregularly, over the entire surface.

When is an eruption universal?

When the whole integument is involved, without any intervening healthy skin.

When is an eruption said to be discrete?

When the lesions constituting the eruption are isolated, having more or less intervening normal skin.

When is an eruption confluent?

When the lesions constituting the eruption are so closely crowded that a solid sheet results.

When is an eruption uniform?

When the lesions constituting the eruption are all of one type or character.

When is an eruption multiform?

When the lesions constituting the eruption are of two or more types or characters.

When are lesions said to be aggregated?

When they tend to form groups or closely-crowded patches.

When are lesions disseminated?

When they are irregularly scattered, with no tendency to form groups or patches.

When is a patch of eruption said to be circinate?

When it presents a rounded form, and usually tending to clear in the centre; as, for example, a patch of ringworm.

When is a patch of eruption said to be annular?

When it is ring-shaped, the central portion being clear; as, for example, in erythema annulare.

What meaning is conveyed by the term "iris"?

The patch of eruption is made up of several concentric rings. Difference of duration of the individual rings, usually slight, tends to give the patch variegated coloration; as, for example, in erythema iris and herpes iris. [Pg 26]

What meaning is conveyed by the term "marginate"?

The sheet of eruption is sharply defined against the healthy skin; as, for example, in erythema marginatum, eczema marginatum.

What meaning is conveyed by the qualifying term "circumscribed"?

The term is applied to small, usually more or less rounded, patches, when sharply defined; as, for example, the typical patches of psoriasis.

When is the qualifying term "gyrate" employed?

When the patches arrange themselves in an irregular winding or festoon-like manner; as, for instance, in some cases of psoriasis. It results, usually, from the coalescence of several rings, the eruption disappearing at the points of contact.

When is an eruption said to be serpiginous?

When the eruption spreads at the border, clearing up at the older part; as, for instance, in the serpiginous syphiloderm.

RELATIVE FREQUENCY.

Name the more common cutaneous diseases and state approximately their frequency.

Eczema, 30.4%; syphilis cutanea, 11.2%; acne, 7.3%; pediculosis, 4%; psoriasis, 3.3%; ringworm, 3.2%; dermatitis, 2.6%; scabies, 2.6%; urticaria, 2.5%; pruritus, 2.1%; seborrhœa, 2.1%; herpes simplex,

1.7%; favus, 1.7%; impetigo, 1.4%; herpes zoster, 1.2%; verruca, 1.1%; tinea versicolor, 1%. Total: eighteen diseases, representing 81 per cent. of all cases met with.

(These percentages are based upon statistics, public and private, of the American Dermatological Association, covering a period of ten years. In private practice the proportion of cases of pediculosis, scabies, favus, and impetigo is much smaller, while acne, acne rosacea, seborrhœa, epithelioma, and lupus are relatively more frequent.) [Pg 27]

CONTAGIOUSNESS.

Name the more actively contagious skin diseases.

Impetigo contagiosa, ringworm, favus, scabies and pediculosis; excluding the exanthemata, erysipelas, syphilis and certain rare and doubtful diseases.

[At the present time when most diseases are presumed to be due to bacteria or parasites the belief in contagiousness, under certain conditions, has considerably broadened.]

RAPIDITY OF CURE.

Is the rapid cure of a skin disease fraught with any danger to the patient?

No. It was formerly so considered, especially by the public and general profession, and the impression still holds to some extent, but it is not in accord with dermatological experience.

OINTMENT BASES.

Name the several fats in common use for ointment bases.

Lard, petrolatum (or cosmoline or vaseline), cold cream and lanolin.

State the relative advantages of these several bases.

Lard is the best all-around base, possessing penetrating properties scarcely exceeded by any other fat.

Petrolatum is also valuable, having little, if any, tendency to change; it is useful as a protective, but is lacking in its power of penetration.

Cold Cream (ungt. aquæ rosæ) is soothing and cooling, and may often be used when other fatty applications disagree.

Lanolin is said to surpass in its power of penetration all other bases, but this is not borne out by experience. It is an unsatisfactory base when used alone. It should be mixed with another base in about the proportion of 25% to 50%.

These several bases may, and often with advantage, be variously combined. [Pg 28]

What is to be added to these several bases if a stiffer ointment is required?

Simple cerate, wax, spermaceti, or suet; or in some instances, a pulverulent substance, such as starch, boric acid, and zinc oxide.

CLASS I.—DISORDERS OF THE GLANDS.

Hyperidrosis.

Fig. 6.

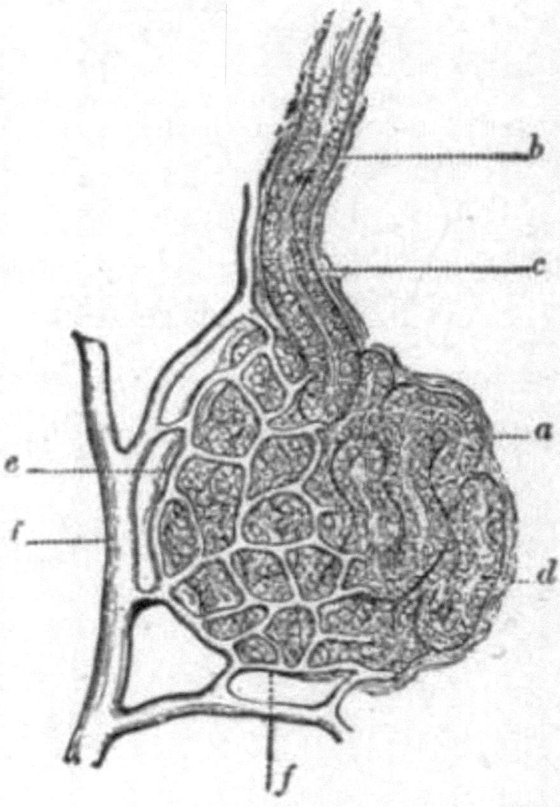

A normal sweat-gland, highly magnified. *(After Neumann.)*

a, Sweat-coil: *b*, sweat-duct; *c*, lumen of duct; *d*, connective-tissue capsule; *e* and *f*, arterial trunk and capillaries.

What is hyperidrosis?

Hyperidrosis is a functional disturbance of the sweat-glands, characterized by an increased production of sweat. This increase may be slight or excessive, local or general. [Pg 29]

As a local affection, what parts are most commonly involved?

The hands, feet, especially the palmar and plantar surfaces, the axillæ and the genitalia.

Describe the symptoms of the local forms of hyperidrosis.

The essential, and frequently the sole symptom, is more or less profuse sweating.

If the hands are the parts involved, they are noted to be wet, clammy and sometimes cold.

If involving the soles, the skin often becomes more or less macerated and sodden in appearance, and as a result of this maceration and continued irritation they may become inflamed, especially about the borders of the affected parts, and present a pinkish or pinkish-red color, having a violaceous tinge. The sweat undergoes change and becomes offensive.

Is hyperidrosis acute or chronic?

Usually chronic, although it may also occur as an acute affection.

What is the etiology of hyperidrosis?

Debility is commonly the cause in general hyperidrosis; the local forms are probably neurotic in origin.

What is the prognosis?

The disease is usually persistent and often rebellious to treatment; in many instances a permanent cure is possible, in others palliation. Relapses are not uncommon.

What systemic remedies are employed in hyperidrosis?

Ergot, belladonna, gallic acid, mineral acids, and tonics. Constitutional treatment is rarely of benefit in the local forms of hyperidrosis, and external applications are seldom of service in general hyperidrosis. Precipitated sulphur, a teaspoonful twice daily, is also well spoken of, combined, if necessary, with an astringent.

What external remedies are employed in the local forms?

Astringent lotions of zinc sulphate, tannin and alum, applied several times daily, with or without the supplementary use of dusting-powders. Weak solutions of formaldehyde, one to one hundred, are sometimes of value. [Pg 30]

Dusting-powders of boric acid and zinc oxide, to which may be added from ten to thirty grains of salicylic acid to the ounce, to be used freely and often:—

> ℞ Pulv. ac. salicylici, ... gr. x-xxx. Pulv. ac. borici, ... ʒv. Pulv. zinci oxidi, ... ʒiij M.

Diachylon ointment, and an ointment containing a drachm of tannin to the ounce; more especially applicable in hyperidrosis of the feet. The parts are first thoroughly washed, rubbed dry with towels and dusting-powder, and the ointment applied on strips of muslin or lint and bound on; the dressing is renewed twice daily, the parts each time being rubbed dry with soft towels and dusting-powder, and the treatment continued for ten days to two weeks, after which the dusting-powder is to be used alone for several weeks. No water is to be used after the first washing until the ointment is discontinued. One such course will occasionally suffice, but not infrequently a repetition is necessary.

Faradization and galvanization are sometimes serviceable. Repeated mild exposures to the Röntgen rays have a favorable influence in some instances.

Sudamen.

(*Synonym:* Miliaria crystallina.)

What is sudamen?

Sudamen is a non-inflammatory disorder of the sweat-glands, characterized by pin-point to pin-head-sized, discrete but thickly-set, superficial, translucent whitish vesicles.

Describe the clinical characters.

The lesions develop rapidly and in great numbers, either irregularly or in crops, and are usually to be seen as discrete, closely-crowded, whitish, or pearl-colored minute elevations, occurring most abundantly upon the trunk. In appearance they resemble minute dew-drops. They are non-inflammatory, without areola, never become purulent, and evince no tendency to rupture, the fluid disappearing by absorption, and the epidermal covering by desquamation. [Pg 31]

Give the course and duration of sudamen.

New crops may appear as the older lesions are disappearing, and the affection persist for some time, or, on the other hand, the whole process may come to an end in several days or a week. In short, the course and duration depend upon the subsidence or persistence of the cause.

What is the anatomical seat of sudamen?

The lesions are formed between the lamellæ of the corneous layer, usually the upper part; and are thought to be due to some change in the character of the epithelial cells of this layer, probably from high temperature, giving rise to a blocking up of the surface outlet.

What is the cause of sudamen?

Debility, especially when associated with high fever. The eruption is often seen in the course of typhus, typhoid and rheumatic fevers.

How would you treat sudamen?

By constitutional remedies directed against the predisposing factor or factors, and the application of cooling lotions of vinegar or alcohol and water, or dusting-powders of starch and lycopodium.

Hydrocystoma.

Describe hydrocystoma.

Hydrocystoma is a cystic affection of the sweat-gland ducts, seated upon the face. The lesions may be present in scant numbers or in more or less profusion. They have the appearance of boiled sago grains imbedded in the skin; the larger lesions may have a bluish color, especially about the periphery. It is not common, and is usually seen in washerwomen and laundresses, or those exposed to moist heat. In some cases it tends to disappear during the winter months. There are no subjective symptoms.

Treatment consists of puncturing the lesions and application of dusting-powder. Avoidance of the exciting cause (moist heat) is important.

Anidrosis.

Describe anidrosis.

It is the opposite condition of hyperidrosis, and is characterized [Pg 32] by diminution or suppression of the sweat secretion. It occurs to some extent in certain systemic diseases and also in some affections of the skin, such as ichthyosis; nerve-injuries may give rise to localized sweat-suppression.

Treatment is based upon general principles; friction, warm and hot-vapor baths, electricity and similar measures are of service.

Bromidrosis.

(*Synonym:* Osmidrosis.)

Describe bromidrosis.

Bromidrosis is a functional disturbance of the sweat-glands characterized by a sweat secretion of an offensive odor. The sweat production may be normal in quantity or more or less excessive, usually the latter. The condition may be local or general, commonly the former. It is closely allied to hyperidrosis, and may often be considered identical, the odor resulting from rapid decomposition of the sweat secretion. The decomposition and resulting odor have been thought due to the presence of bacteria.

What parts are most commonly affected in bromidrosis?

The feet and the axillæ.

What is the treatment of bromidrosis?

It is essentially the same as that of hyperidrosis (*q. v.*), consisting of applications of astringent lotions, dusting-powders, especially those containing boric acid and salicylic acid, and the continuous application of diachylon ointment. In obstinate cases weak formaldehyde solutions, Röntgen rays, and high-frequency currents can be tried.

Chromidrosis.

Describe chromidrosis.

This is a functional disorder of the sweat-glands characterized by a secretion variously colored, and usually increased in quantity. It is, as a rule, limited to a circumscribed area. The most common color is red. The condition is probably of neurotic origin and tends to recur. (True chromidrosis is extremely rare; most of the cases formerly thought to be such are now known to be examples of pseudochromidrosis.) [Pg 33]

Treatment should be invigorating and tonic, with special reference toward the nervous system. The various methods of local electrization should also be resorted to.

Mild antiseptic and astringent lotions or dusting powders should also be advised.

Red chromidrosis or *Pseudochromidrosis* is a condition in which the coloring of the sweat occurs after its excretion and is due to the presence of chromatogenous bacteria which are found attached to the hairs of the part in agglutinated masses. The axilla is the favorite site. Treatment consists of frequent soap-and-water washings, and the application of boric acid, resorcin, and corrosive sublimate lotions.

Uridrosis.

Describe uridrosis.

Uridrosis is a rare condition in which the sweat secretion contains the elements of the urine, especially urea. In marked cases the salt may be noticeable upon the skin as a colorless or whitish crystalline deposit. In most instances it has been preceded or accompanied by partial or complete suppression of the renal functions.

Phosphoridrosis.

Describe phosphoridrosis.

Phosphoridrosis is a rare condition, in which the sweat is phosphorescent. It has been observed in the later stages of phthisis, in miliaria, and in those who have eaten of putrid fish.

Seborrhœa (Eczema Seborrhoicum).

Synonyms: (Steatorrhœa; Acne sebacea; Ichthyosis sebacea; Dandruff.)

What is seborrhœa?

Seborrhœa is a disease of the sebaceous glands, characterized by an excessive and abnormal secretion of sebaceous matter, appearing on the skin as an oily coating, crusts, or scales.

In many cases the sweat-glands are likewise implicated, and the process may also be distinctly, although usually mildly, inflammatory. [Pg 34]

At what age is seborrhœa usually observed?

Between fifteen and forty. It may, however, occur at any age.

Name the parts most commonly affected.

The scalp, face, and (less frequently) the sternal and interscapular regions of the trunk. It is sometimes seen on other parts.

What varieties of seborrhœa are encountered?

Seborrhœa oleosa and seborrhœa sicca; not infrequently the disease is of a mixed type.

What are the symptoms of seborrhœa oleosa?

The sole symptom is an unnatural oiliness, variable as to degree. Its most common sites are the regions of the scalp, nose, and forehead. In many instances mild rosacea coexists with oily seborrhœa of the nose.

Give the symptoms of seborrhœa sicca.

A variable degree of greasy scalines, which may be seated upon a pale, hyperæmic or mildly inflammatory surface.

The parts affected are covered scantily or more or less abundantly with somewhat greasy, grayish, or brownish-gray scales. If upon the scalp (*dandruff, pityriasis capitis*), small particles of scales are found scattered through the hair, and when the latter is brushed or combed, fall over the shoulders. If upon the face, in addition to the scaliness, the sebaceous ducts are usually seen to be enlarged and filled with sebaceous matter.

Describe the symptoms of the ordinary or mixed type.

It is common upon the scalp. The skin is covered with irregularly diffused, greasy, grayish or brownish scales and crusts, in some cases moderate in quantity, in others so great that large irregular masses are formed, pasting the hair to the scalp. If removed, the scales and crusts rapidly re-form. The skin beneath is found slate-colored, hyperæmic or mildly inflammatory, and exceptionally it has in places an eczematous aspect (*eczema seborrhoicum*). Extraneous matter, such as dust and dirt, collects upon the parts, and the whole mass may become more or less offensive. There is a strong tendency to falling-out of the hair. Itching may or may not be present.

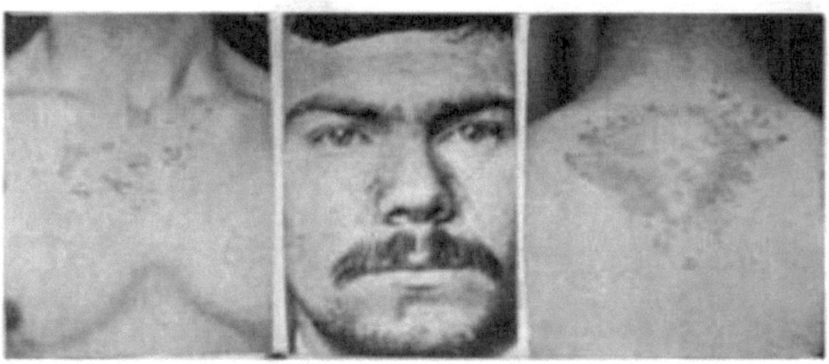

Seborrhœa (Eczema Seborrhoicum).

[Pg 35]

Describe the symptoms of seborrhœa of the trunk and other parts.

Fig. 7.

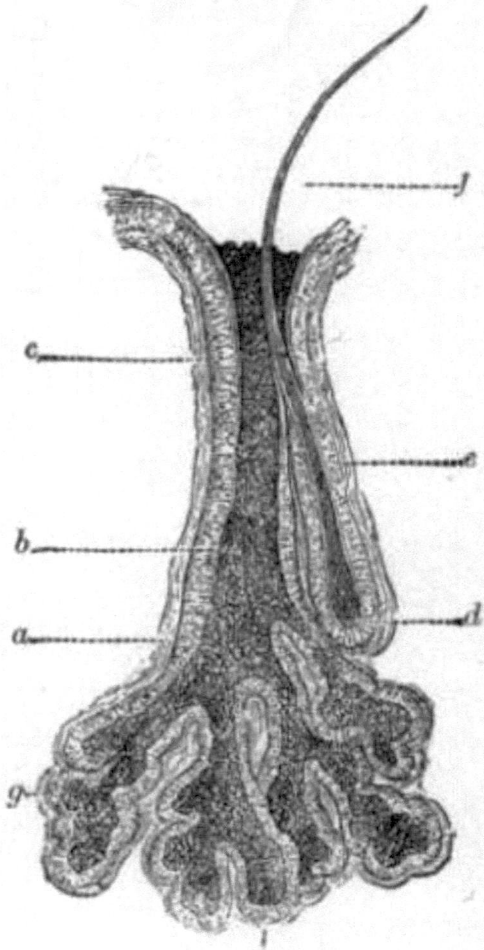

A normal sebaceous gland in connection with a lanugo hair. (*After Neumann.*)

a, Capsule; *b*, fatty secretion; *c*, *h*, secreting cells; *d*, root of lanugo hair; *e*, hair-sac; *f*, hair-shaft; *g*, acini of sebaceous gland.

Seborrhœa corporis differs in a measure, in its symptoms, from seborrhœa of the scalp and is usually illustrative of the variety known as eczema seborrhoicum; it occurs as one or several irregular or circinate, slightly hyperæmic or moderately inflammatory patches, covered with dirty or grayish-looking greasy scales or crusts, usually moderate in quantity, and upon removal are found to have projections into the sebaceous ducts. It is commonly seen upon the sternal and interscapular regions. It rarely exists independently in these regions, being usually associated with and following the disease on the scalp. It may also invade the axillæ, genitocrural, and other regions. [Pg 36]

What is the usual course of seborrhœa?

Essentially chronic, the disease varying in intensity from time to time. In occasional instances it disappears spontaneously.

Give the cause or causes of seborrhœa.

General debility, anæmia, chlorosis, dyspepsia, and similar conditions are to be variously looked upon as predisposing.

In some instances, however, the disease seems to be purely local in character, and to be entirely independent of any constitutional or predisposing condition. The view recently advanced that the disease is of parasitic nature and contagious has been steadily gaining ground.

What is the pathology of seborrhœa?

Seborrhœa is a disease of the sebaceous glands, and probably often involving the sweat-glands also; its products, as found upon the skin, consisting of the sebaceous secretion, epithelial cells from the glands and ducts, and more or less extraneous matter. Not infrequently evidences of superficial inflammatory action are also to be found, and it is especially for this type that the name eczema seborrhoicum is most appropriate. In long-continued and neglected cases slight atrophy of the gland-structures may occur.

With what diseases are you likely to confound seborrhœa?

Upon the scalp, with eczema and psoriasis; upon the face, with lupus erythematosus and eczema; and upon the trunk, with psoriasis and ringworm.

As a rule, the clinical features of seborrhœa are sufficiently characteristic to prevent error.

What are the differential points?

Eczema, psoriasis, and lupus erythematosus are diseases in which there are distinct *inflammatory symptoms*, such as thickening and infiltration and redness; moreover, psoriasis, and this holds true as to ringworm also, occurs in sharply-defined, circumscribed patches, and lupus erythematosus has a peculiar violaceous tint and an elevated and marginate border. A microscopic examination of the epidermic scrapings would be of crucial value in differentiating from ringworm.

Quite frequently, especially in the interscapular and sternal regions, the segmental configuration constitutes an important feature of seborrhœa—of the eczema seborrhoicum variety. [Pg 37]

What is the prognosis in seborrhœa?

Favorable. All types are curable, and when upon the non-hairy regions, usually readily so; upon the scalp it is often obstinate. Relapses are not uncommon.

In those cases of seborrhœa capitis which have been long-continued or neglected, and attended with loss of hair, this loss may be more or less permanent, although ordinarily much can be done to promote a regrowth (see *Treatment of Alopecia*).

How would you treat seborrhœa of the scalp?

By constitutional (if indicated) and local remedies; the former having in view correction or modification of the predisposing factor or factors, and the latter removal of the sebaceous accumulations and the application of mildly stimulating antiseptic ointments or lotions.

What constitutional remedies are commonly employed?

The various tonics, such as iron, quinine, strychnia, cod-liver oil, arsenic, the vegetable bitters, laxatives, malt and similar preparations. The line of treatment is to be based upon indications.

How do you free the scalp of the sebaceous accumulations?

In mild types of the disease shampooing with simple Castile soap (or any other good toilet soap) and hot water will suffice; in those cases in which there is considerable scale-and crust-formation the tincture of green soap (tinct. saponis viridis) is to be employed in place of the toilet soap, and in some of these latter cases it may be necessary to soften the crusts with a previous soaking with olive oil.

The frequency of the shampoo depends upon the conditions. In mild cases once in five or ten days will be sufficiently frequent to keep the parts clean, but in those cases in which there is rapid scale- or crust-production once daily or every second day may at first be demanded.

Name the most effectual applications in seborrhœa capitis.

Sulphur, ammoniated mercury, salicylic acid, resorcin, and carbolic acid.

Sulphur is used in the form of an ointment, from twenty grains to one drachm in the ounce. Ammoniated mercury, in the form of an ointment, ten to sixty grains to the ounce. Salicylic acid, either alone as an ointment, ten to thirty grains to the ounce; or it may [Pg 38]

often be added with advantage, in the same proportion, to the sulphur or ammoniated mercury ointment above named. Resorcin, either as an ointment, ten to thirty grains to the ounce, or as an alcoholic or aqueous lotion, as the following:—

℞ Resorcini, ... ʒj-ʒiss. Ol. ricini,
.... ♏xxx-fʒij. Alcoholis,
.... f℥iv. M.

Carbolic acid, to the amount of ten to thirty grains, can be added to this. If an aqueous lotion is desirable, then in the above formula the oleum ricini is replaced with glycerine, and the alcohol with water; three to five minims of glycerine in each ounce is usually sufficient, as a greater quantity makes the resulting lotion sticky.

Petrolatum alone, or with 10 to 30 per cent. lanolin, is usually the most satisfactory base for the ointments. In some cases of the inflammatory variety the skin is found quite irritable, and the mildest applications are at first only admissible.

How are the remedies to be applied?

A small quantity of the lotion, ointment, or oil is gently applied to the skin; when to the scalp, a lotion or oil can be conveniently applied by means of an eye-dropper. In the beginning of the treatment an application once or twice daily is ordered; later, as the disease becomes less active, once every second or third day.

How is seborrhœa upon other parts to be treated?

In the same general manner as seborrhœa of the scalp, except that the local applications must be somewhat weaker. The several sulphur lotions employed in the treatment of acne (*q. v.*) may also be used when the disease is upon these parts. In obstinate patchy cases occasional paintings with a 20 to 50 per cent alcoholic solution of resorcin is curative; following the painting a mild salve should be used.

Comedo.

(*Synonyms:* Blackheads; Flesh-worms.)

What is comedo?

Comedo is a disorder of the sebaceous glands, characterized by yellowish or blackish pin-point or pin-head-sized puncta or elevations corresponding to the gland-orifices. [Pg 39]

At what age and upon what parts are comedones found?

Usually between fifteen and thirty, and upon the face and upper part of the trunk, where they may exist sparsely or in great numbers. They are occasionally associated with oily seborrhœa, the parts presenting a greasy or soiled appearance.

Exceptionally they occur as distinct, and usually symmetrical, groups upon the forehead or the cheeks. On the upper trunk so-called double and multiple comedo have been noted—the two, three, or even four closely-contiguous blackheads are, beneath the surface, intercommunicable, the dividing duct-walls having apparently disappeared by fusion.

Describe an individual lesion.

It is pin-point to pin-head in size, dark yellowish, and usually with a central blackish point (hence the name *blackheads*). There is scarcely perceptible elevation, unless the amount of retained secretion is excessive. Upon pressure this may be ejected, the small, rounded orifice through which it is expressed giving it a thread-like shape (hence the name *flesh-worms*).

What is the usual course of comedo?

Chronic. The lesions may persist indefinitely or the condition may be somewhat variable. In many instances, either as a result of pressure or in consequence of chemical change in the sebaceous plugs or of the addition of a microbic factor, inflammation is excited and acne results. The two conditions are, in fact, usually associated.

Fig. 8.

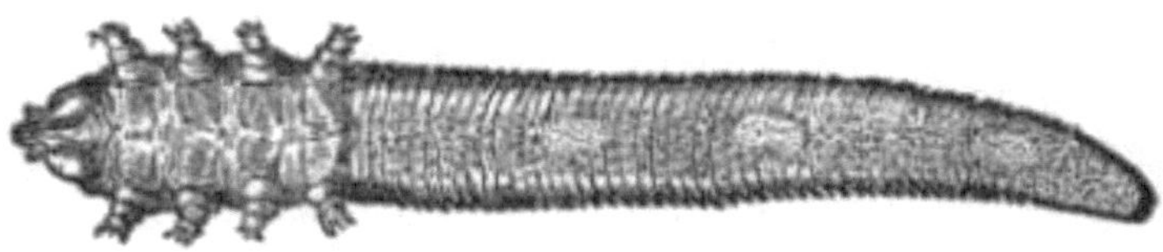

Demodex Folliculorum, X 300. Ventral surface. (*After Simon*).

To what may comedo often be ascribed?

To disorders of digestion, constipation, chlorosis, menstrual disturbance, lack of tone in the muscular fibres of the skin, the infrequent use of soap, and working in a dirty or dusty atmosphere. [Pg 40] A small parasite (*demodex folliculorum, acarus folliculorum*) is sometimes found in the sebaceous mass, but its presence is without etiological significance, as it is also found in healthy follicles. A microbacillus has been found by several observers, and credited with etiological influence.

What is the pathology of comedo?

The sebaceous ducts or glands, or both, become blocked up with retained secretion and epithelial cells. The dark points which usually mark the lesions are probably due to accumulation of dirt, but may, as some writers maintain, be due to the presence of pigment-granules resulting from chemical change in the sebaceous matter.

Is there any difficulty in the diagnosis of comedo?

No. It can scarcely be confounded with milium, as in this latter disease the lesion has no open outlet, no black point, and the contents cannot be squeezed out.

Give the prognosis of comedo.

The result of treatment is usually favorable, although the disease is often rebellious. Relapses are not uncommon.

How would you treat a case of comedo?

By systemic (if indicated) and local measures.

The constitutional treatment aims at correction or palliation of the predisposing conditions, and the external applications have in view a removal of the sebaceous plugs and stimulation of the glands and skin to healthy action.

Fig. 9.

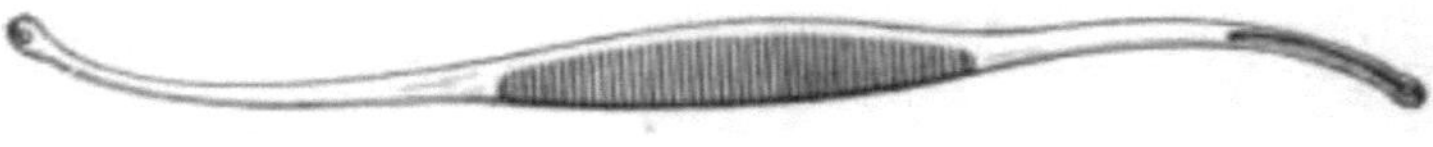

Comedo Extractor.

Name the systemic remedies commonly employed.

Cod-liver oil, iron, quinine, arsenic, nux vomica and other tonics; ergot in those cases in which there is lack of muscular tone, salines and aperient pills in constipation. The digestion is to be looked after and the bowels kept regular; indigestible food of all kinds is to be interdicted. Hygienic measures, such as general and local bathing, local massage, calisthenics, and open-air exercise, are of service. [Pg 41]

Describe the local treatment.

Steaming the face or prolonged applications of hot water; washing with ordinary toilet soap and hot water, or, in sluggish cases, using tincture of green soap (tinct. saponis viridis) instead of the toilet soap; removal of the sebaceous plugs by mechanical means, such as lateral pressure with the finger ends or perpendicular pressure with a watch-key with rounded edges, or with an instrument specially contrived for this purpose; and after these preliminary measures, which should be carried out every night, a stimulating sulphur ointment or lotion, such as employed in the treatment of acne (*q. v.*), is to be thoroughly applied. The following is valuable:—

> ℞ Zinci sulphatis, Potassi sulphureti, ...āā......... ʒj-ʒiv.
> Alcoholi .... f℥ss. Aquæ, ...
> q.s. ad. ...... f℥iv. M.

Should slight scaliness or a mild degree of irritation of the skin be brought about, active external treatment is to be discontinued for a few days and soothing applications made. Resorcin, in lotion, 3 to 25 per cent strength, is through the exfoliation it provokes, frequently of value; the resorcin paste referred to in acne can also be used for this purpose.

Moderately strong applications of the Faradic current, repeated once or twice weekly, are sometimes of service; also weak to moderately strong applications of the continuous and high-frequency currents. Röntgen-ray treatment can also be resorted to in extremely obstinate cases.

In occasional instances sulphur preparations not only fail to do good, but materially aggravate the condition. In such cases, if resorcin preparations also fail, the mercurial lotion and ointment employed in acne may be prescribed. Mercurial and sulphur applications should not be used, it need scarcely be said, within a week or ten days of each other, otherwise an increase in the comedones and a slight darkening of the skin result from the formation of the black sulphuret of mercury. [Pg 42]

Milium.

(*Synonyms:* Grutum; Strophulus Albidus.)

What is milium?

Milium consists in the formation of small, whitish or yellowish, rounded, pearly, non-inflammatory elevations situated in the upper part of the corium.

Describe the clinical appearances.

The lesions are usually pin-head in size, whitish or yellowish, seemingly more or less translucent, rounded or acuminated, without aperture or duct, are superficially seated in the skin, and project slightly above the surface.

They appear about the face, especially about the eyelids; they may occur also, although rarely, upon other parts. But one or several may be present, or they may exist in numbers.

What is the course of milium?

The lesions develop slowly, and may then remain stationary for years. Their presence gives rise to no disturbance, and, unless they are large in size or exist in numbers, causes but slight disfigurement.

Fig. 10.

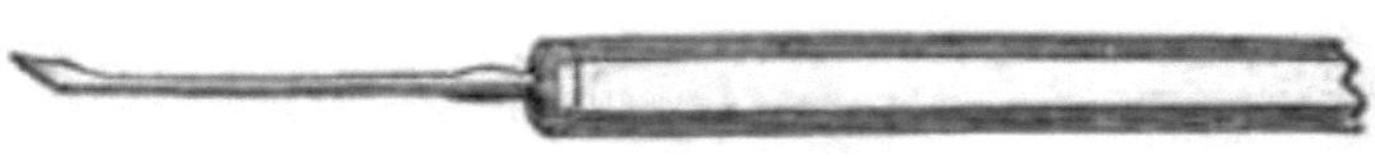

Milium Needle.

In rare instances they may undergo calcareous metamorphosis, constituting the so-called *cutaneous calculi*.

What is the anatomical seat of milium?

The sebaceous gland (probably one or several of the superficially-situated acini), the duct of which is in some manner obliterated, the sebaceous matter collects, becomes inspissated and calcareous, forming the pin-head lesion. The epidermis is the external covering.

What is the treatment?

The usual plan is to prick or incise each lesion and press out the contents. In some milia it may be necessary also, in order to prevent a return, to touch the base of the excavation with tincture of [Pg 43] iodine or with silver nitrate. Electrolysis is also effectual. In those cases where the lesions are numerous the production of exfoliation of the epiderm by means of resorcin applications (see acne) is a good plan.

Steatoma.

(*Synonyms:* Sebaceous Cyst; Sebaceous Tumor; Wen.)

Describe steatoma.

Steatoma, or sebaceous cyst, appears as a variously-sized, elevated, rounded or semi-globular, soft or firm tumor, freely movable and painless, and having its seat in the corium or subcutaneous tissue. The overlying skin is normal in color, or it may be whitish or pale from distention; in some a gland-duct orifice may be seen, but, as a rule, this is absent.

What are the favorite regions for the development of steatoma?

The scalp, face and back. One or several may be present.

What is the course of sebaceous cysts?

Their growth is slow, and, after attaining a variable size, may remain stationary. They may exist indefinitely without causing any inconvenience beyond the disfigurement. Exceptionally, in enormously distended growths, suppuration and ulceration result.

What is the pathology?

A steatoma is a cyst of the sebaceous gland and duct, produced by retained secretion. The contents may be hard and friable, soft and cheesy, or even fluid, of a grayish, whitish or yellowish color, and with or without a fetid odor; the mass consisting of fat-drops, epidermic cells, cholesterin, and sometimes hairs.

Are sebaceous cysts likely to be confounded with gummata?

No. Gummata grow more rapidly, are usually painful to the touch, are not freely movable, and tend to break down and ulcerate.

Describe the treatment of steatoma.

A linear incision is made, and the mass and enveloping sac [Pg 44] dissected out. If the sac is permitted to remain, reproduction almost invariably takes place.

CLASS II.—INFLAMMATIONS.

Erythema Simplex.

What do you understand by erythema simplex?

Erythema simplex is a hyperæmic disorder characterized by redness, occurring in the form of variously-sized and shaped, diffused or circumscribed, non-elevated patches.

Name the two general classes into which the simple erythemata are divided.

Idiopathic and symptomatic.

What do you include in the idiopathic class?

Those erythemas due to external causes, such as cold and heat (*erythema caloricum*), the action of the sun (*erythema solare*), traumatism (*erythema traumaticum*), and the various poisons or chemical irritants (*erythema venenatum*).

What do you include in the symptomatic class?

Those rashes often preceding or accompanying certain of the systemic diseases, and those due to disorders of the digestive tract, stomachic and intestinal toxins, to the ingestion of certain drugs, and to use of the therapeutic serums.

Describe the symptoms of erythema simplex.

The essential symptom is redness—simple hyperæmia—without elevation or infiltration, disappearing under pressure, and sometimes attended by slight heat or burning; it may be patchy or diffused. In the idiopathic class, if the cause is continued, dermatitis may result.

What is to be said about the distribution of the simple erythemata?

The idiopathic rashes, as inferred from the nature of the causes, are usually limited.

The symptomatic erythemas are more or less generalized; desquamation sometimes follows. [Pg 45]

Describe the treatment of the simple erythemata.

A removal of the cause in idiopathic rashes is all that is needed, the erythema sooner or later subsiding. The same may be stated of the symptomatic erythemata, but in these there is at times difficulty in recognizing the etiological factor; constitutional treatment, if necessary, is to be based upon general principles. Intestinal antiseptics are useful in some instances.

Local treatment, which is rarely needed, consists of the use of dusting-powders or mild cooling and astringent lotions, such as are employed in the treatment of acute eczema (q. v.).

Erythema Intertrigo.

(*Synonym:* Chafing.)

What do you understand by erythema intertrigo?

Erythema intertrigo is a hyperæmic disorder occurring on parts where the natural folds of the skin come in contact, and is characterized by redness, to which may be added an abraded surface and maceration of the epidermis.

Describe the symptoms of erythema intertrigo.

The skin of the involved region gradually becomes hyperæmic, but is without elevation or infiltration; a feeling of heat and soreness is usually experienced. If the condition continue, the increased perspiration and moisture of the parts give rise to maceration of the epidermis and a mucoid discharge; actual inflammation may eventually result.

What is the course of erythema intertrigo?

The affection may pass away in a few days or persist several weeks, the duration depending, in a great measure, upon the cause.

Mention the causes of erythema intertrigo.

The causes are usually local. It is seen chiefly in children, especially in fat subjects, in whom friction and moisture of contiguous parts of the body, usually the region of the neck, buttocks and genitalia, are more common; in such, uncleanliness or the too free use of soap washings will often act as the exciting factor. Disorders of [Pg 46] the stomach or intestinal canal apparently have a predisposing influence.

What treatment would you advise in erythema intertrigo?

The folds or parts are to be kept from contact by means of lint or absorbent cotton; thin, flat bags of cheese cloth or similar material partly filled with dusting-powder, and kept clean by frequent changes, are excellent for this purpose, and usually curative. Cleanliness is essential, but it is to be kept within the bounds of common sense. Dusting-powders and cooling and astringent lotions, such as are employed in the treatment of acute eczema (*q. v.*), can also be advised. The following lotion is valuable:—

℞ Pulv. calaminæ, Pulv. zinci oxidi, ...āā......... ʒiss.
Glycerinæ, ... ♏xxx Alcoholis,
.... fʒij Aquæ, ...
Oss. M.

Exceptionally a mild ointment, alone or supplementary to a lotion, acts more satisfactorily.

In persistent or obstinate cases attention should also be directed to the state of the general health, especially as regards the digestive tract.

Erythema Multiforme.

What is erythema multiforme?

Erythema multiforme is an acute, inflammatory disease, characterized by reddish, more or less variegated macules, papules, and tubercles, occurring as discrete lesions or in patches of various size and shape.

Upon what parts of the body does the eruption appear?

Usually upon the extremities, especially the dorsal aspect, from the knees and elbows down, and about the face and neck; it may, however, be more or less general.

Describe the symptoms of erythema multiforme.

With or without precursory symptoms of malaise, gastric uneasiness or rheumatic pains, the eruption suddenly makes its appearance, [Pg 47] assuming an erythematous, papular, tubercular or mixed character; as a rule, one type of lesion predominates. The lesions tend to increase in size and intensity, remain stationary for several days or a week, and then gradually fade; during this time there may have been outbreaks of new lesions. In color they are pink, red, or violaceous. Slight itching may or may not be present. Exceptionally, in general cases, the eruption partakes of the nature of both urticaria and erythema multiforme, and itching may be quite a decided symptom. In some instances there is preceding and accompanying febrile action, usually slight in character; in others there may be some rheumatic swelling of one or more joints.

Fig. 11.

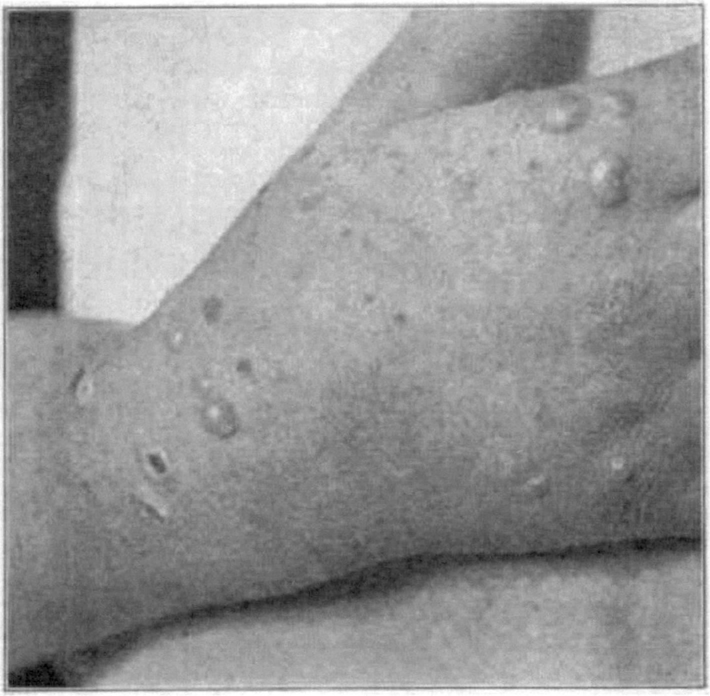

Erythema Multiforme, in which many of the lesions have become bullous—

Erythema Bullosum.

[Pg 48]

What type of the eruption is most common?

The papular, appearing usually upon the backs of the hands and forearms, and not infrequently, also, upon the face, legs and feet. The papules are usually pea-sized, flattened, and of a dark red or violaceous color.

Describe the various shapes which the erythematous lesions may assume.

Often the patches are distinctly ring-shaped, with a clear centre—*erythema annulare*; or they are made up of several concentric rings, presenting variegated coloring—*erythema iris*; or a more or less extensive patch may spread with a sharply-defined border, the older part tending to fade—*erythema marginatum*; or several rings may coalesce, with a disappearance of the coalescing parts, and serpentine lines or bands result—*erythema gyratum*.

Does the eruption of erythema multiforme ever assume a vesicular or bullous character?

Yes. In exceptional instances, the inflammatory process may be sufficiently intense to produce vesiculation, usually at the summits of the papules—*erythema vesiculosum*; and in some instances, blebs may be formed—*erythema bullosum*. A vesicular or bullous lesion may become immediately surrounded by a ring-like vesicle or bleb, and outside of this another form; a patch may be made up of as many as several such rings—*herpes iris*. In the vesicular and bullous cases the lips and the mucous membranes of the mouth and nose also may be the seat of similar lesions.

What is the course of erythema multiforme?

Acute, the symptoms disappearing spontaneously, usually in one to three or four weeks. In some instances the recurrences take place so rapidly that the disease assumes a chronic aspect; it is possible that such cases are midway cases between this disease and dermatitis herpetiformis.

Mention the etiological factors in erythema multiforme.

The causes are obscure. Digestive disturbance, rheumatic conditions, and the ingestion of certain drugs are at times influential. Intestinal toxins are doubtless important etiological factors in some cases. Certain foods, such as are apt to undergo rapid putrefactive [Pg 49] or fermentative change, especially pork meats, oysters, fish, crabs, lobsters, etc., are, therefore, not infrequently of apparent causative influence. It is most frequently observed in spring and autumn months, and in early adult life. The disease is not uncommon.

What is the pathology of erythema multiforme?

It is a mildly inflammatory disorder, somewhat similar to urticaria, and presumably due to vasomotor disturbance; the amount of exudation, which is variable, determines the character of the lesions.

Name the diagnostic points of erythema multiforme.

The multiformity of the eruption, the size of the papules, often its limitation to certain parts, its course and the entire or comparative absence of itching.

It resembles urticaria at times, but the lesions of this latter disease are evanescent, disappearing and reappearing usually in the most capricious manner, are commonly seated about the trunk, and are exceedingly itchy.

In the vesicular and bullous types the acute character of the outbreak, the often segmental and ring-like shape, their frequent origin from erythematous papules, and the distribution and association with the more common manifestations, are always suggestive.

What prognosis would you give in erythema multiforme?

Always favorable; the eruption usually disappears in ten days to three weeks, although in rare instances new crops may appear from day to day or week to week, and the process last one or two months. One or more recurrences in succeeding years are not uncommon. Those rare cases in which vesicular or bullous lesions are also seen on the lips and in the mouth, are more prone to longer duration and to more frequent recurrences.

What remedies are commonly prescribed in erythema multiforme?

Quinin, and, if constipation is present, saline laxatives. Calcined magnesia is valuable as a laxative. Intestinal antiseptics, such as salol, thymol, and sodium salicylate, are valuable in cases probably due to intestinal toxins. In those exceptional instances in which there may be associated febrile action and rheumatic swelling of the joints, the patient should be kept in bed till these symptoms [Pg 50] subside. Local applications are rarely required, but in those exceptional cases in which itching or burning is present, cooling lotions of alcohol and water or vinegar and water are to be prescribed. The vesicular and bullous types demand mild protective applications, such as used in eczema and pemphigus.

Erythema Nodosum.

(*Synonym:* Dermatitis contusiformis.)

What is erythema nodosum?

Erythema nodosum is an inflammatory affection, of an acute type, characterized by the formation of variously-sized, roundish, more or less elevated erythematous nodes.

Is there any special region of predilection for the eruption of erythema nodosum?

Yes. The tibial surfaces, to which the eruption is often limited; not infrequently, however, other parts may be involved, more especially the arms and forearms.

Describe the symptoms of erythema nodosum.

The eruption makes its appearance suddenly, and is usually ushered in with febrile disturbance, gastric uneasiness, malaise, and rheumatic pains and swelling about the joints. The lesions vary in size from a cherry to a hen's egg, are rounded or ovalish, tender and painful, have a glistening and tense look, and are of a bright red, erysipelatous color which merges gradually into the sound skin. At first they are somewhat hard, but later they soften and appear as if about to break down, but this, however, never occurs, absorption invariably taking place. In occasional instances they are hemorrhagic. Exceptionally the lesions of erythema multiforme are also present. Lymphangitis is sometimes observed. In rare instances symptoms pointing to visceral involvement, to cerebral invasion, and to heart complications have been observed.

Are the lesions in erythema nodosum usually numerous?

No. As a rule not more than five to twenty nodes are present.

What is the course of erythema nodosum?

Acute. The disease terminating usually in one to three weeks. [Pg 51] As the lesions are disappearing they present the various changes of color observed in an ordinary bruise.

What is known in regard to the etiology?

The affection is closely allied to erythema multiforme, and is, indeed, by some considered a form of that disease. It occurs most frequently in children and young adults, and usually in the spring and autumn months. Intestinal toxins are thought responsible in some cases. Digestive disturbance and rheumatic pain and swellings are often associated with it. By many the malady is thought to be a specific infection.

What is the pathology of erythema nodosum?

The disease is to be viewed as an inflammatory œdema, probably resulting, in some instances at least, from an inflammation of the lymphatics or an embolism of the cutaneous vessels.

What diseases may erythema nodosum resemble?

Bruises, abscesses, and gummata.

How are the lesions of erythema nodosum to be distinguished from these several conditions?

By the bright red or rosy tint, the apparently violent character of the process, the number, situation and course of the lesions.

State the prognosis of erythema nodosum.

Favorable, recovery usually taking place in ten days to several weeks.

State the treatment to be advised in erythema nodosum.

Rest, relative or absolute, depending upon the severity of the case, and an unstimulating diet; internally intestinal antiseptics, quinin and saline laxatives, and locally applications of lead-water and laudanum.

Erythema Induratum.

(*Synonym:* Erythema induratum scrofulosorum.)

What do you understand by erythema induratum?

A rare disease characterized in the beginning by one or more usually deep-seated nodules, and, as a rule, seated in the legs, [Pg 52] especially the calf region. The nodules gradually enlarge, the skin becomes reddish, violaceous or livid in color. Absorption may take place slowly, or the indurations may break down, resulting in an indolent, rather deep-seated ulcer, closely resembling a gummatous ulcer. The disease is slow and persistent, and is commonly met with in girls and young women, usually of strumous type. It suggests a tuberculous origin.

Treatment consists in administration of cod-liver oil, phosphorus and other tonics. Rest is of service. Locally antiseptic applications, and support with roller bandage are to be advised.

Urticaria.

(*Synonyms:* Hives; Nettlerash.)

Give a definition of urticaria.

Urticaria is an inflammatory affection characterized by evanescent whitish, pinkish or reddish elevations, or wheals, variable as to size and shape, and attended by itching, stinging or pricking sensations.

Describe the symptoms of urticaria.

The eruption, erythematous in character and consisting of isolated pea or bean-sized elevations or of linear streaks or irregular patches, limited or more or less general, and usually intensely itchy, makes its appearance suddenly, with or without symptoms of preceding gastric derangement. The lesions are soft or firm, reddish or pinkish-white, with the peripheral portion of a bright red color, and are fugacious in character, disappearing and reappearing in the most capricious manner. In many cases simply drawing the finger over the skin will bring out irregular and linear wheals. In exceptional cases this peculiar property is so pronounced and constant that at any time letters and other symbols may be produced at will, even when such subjects are free from the ordinary urticarial lesions (*urticaria factitia, dermatographism, autographism*).

The mucous membrane of the mouth and throat may also be the seat of wheals and urticarial swellings.

What is the ordinary course of urticaria?

Acute. The disease is usually at an end in several hours or days. [Pg 53]

Does urticaria always pursue an acute course?

No. In exceptional instances the disease is chronic, in the sense that new lesions continue to appear and disappear irregularly from time to time for months or several years, the skin rarely being entirely free (*chronic urticaria*).

Fig. 12.

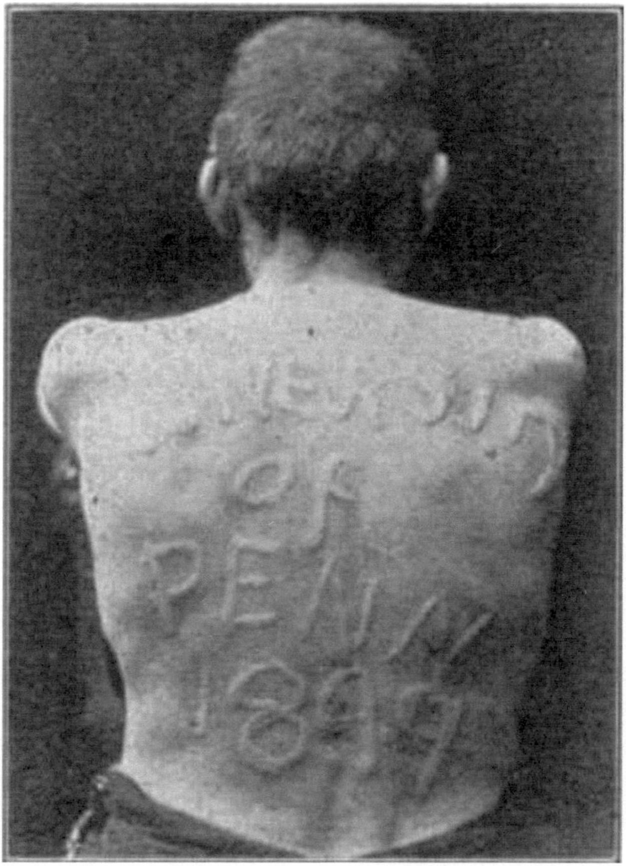

Dermatographism. (*After C.N. Davis.*)

Are subjective symptoms always present in urticaria?

Yes. Itching is commonly a conspicuous symptom, although at times pricking, stinging or a feeling of burning constitutes the chief sensation.

In what way may the eruption be atypical?

Exceptionally the wheals, or lesions, are peculiar as to formation, or another condition or disease may be associated, hence the varieties known as urticaria papulosa, urticaria hæmorrhagica, urticaria tuberosa, and urticaria bullosa.

Describe urticaria papulosa.

Urticaria papulosa (formerly called *lichen urticatus*) is a variety in [Pg 54] which the lesions are small and papular, developing usually out of the ordinary wheals. They appear as a rule suddenly, rarely in great numbers, are scattered, and after a few hours or, more commonly, days gradually disappear. The itching is intense, and in consequence their apices are excoriated. Sometimes the papules are capped with a small vesicle (vesicular urticaria). It is seen more particularly in ill-cared for and badly-nourished young children.

Describe urticaria hæmorrhagica.

Urticaria hæmorrhagica is characterized by lesions similar to ordinary wheals, except that they are somewhat hemorrhagic, partaking, in fact, of the nature of both urticaria and purpura.

Describe urticaria tuberosa.

In urticaria tuberosa the lesions, instead of being pea- or bean-sized, as in typical urticaria, are large and node-like (also called *giant urticaria*).

What is acute-circumscribed œdema?

In rare instances there occurs, along with the ordinary lesions of the disease or as its sole manifestation, sudden and evanescent swelling of the eyelids, ears, lips, tongue, hands, fingers, or feet (*urticaria œdematosa, acute circumscribed œdema, angioneurotic œdema*). One or several of these parts only may be affected at the one attack; in recurrences, so usual in this variety, the same or other parts may exhibit the manifestation.

(These œdematous swellings occurring alone might be looked upon, as they are by most observers, as an independent affection, but its close relationship to ordinary urticaria is often evident.)

Describe urticaria bullosa.

Urticaria bullosa is a variety in which the inflammatory action has been sufficiently great to give rise to fluid exudation, the wheals resulting in the formation of blebs.

What is the etiology of urticaria?

Any irritation from disease, functional or organic, of any internal organ, may give rise to the eruption in those predisposed. Gastric derangement from indigestible or peculiar articles of food, intestinal toxins, and the ingestion of certain drugs are often provocative. The so-called "shell-fish" group of foods play an important etiological part in some cases. Idiosyncrasy to certain articles of food is [Pg 55] also responsible in occasional instances. Various rheumatic and nervous disorders are not infrequently associated with it, and are doubtless of etiological significance. External irritants, also, in predisposed subjects, are at times responsible.

What is the pathology of urticaria?

Anatomically a wheal is seen to be a more or less firm elevation consisting of a circumscribed or somewhat diffused collection of semi-fluid material in the upper layers of the skin. The vasomotor nervous system is probably the main factor in its production; dilatation following spasm of the vessels results in effusion, and in consequence, the overfilled vessels of the central portion are emptied by pressure of the exudation and the central paleness results, while the pressed-back blood gives rise to the bright red periphery.

From what diseases is urticaria to be differentiated?

From erythema simplex, erythema multiforme, erythema nodosum, and erysipelas.

Mention the diagnostic points of urticaria.

The acuteness, character of the lesions, their evanescent nature, the irregular or general distribution, and the intense itching.

What is the prognosis in urticaria?

The acute disease is usually of short duration, disappearing spontaneously or as the result of treatment, in several hours or days; it may recur upon exposure to the exciting cause. The prognosis of chronic urticaria is to be guarded, and will depend upon the ability to discover and remove or modify the predisposing condition.

What systemic measures are to be prescribed in acute urticaria?

Removal of the etiological factor is of first importance. This will be found in most cases to be gastric disturbance from the ingestion of improper or indigestible food, and in such cases a saline purgative is to be given, probably the best for this purpose being the laxative antacid, magnesia; or if the case is severe and food is still in the stomach, an emetic, such as mustard or ipecac, will act more promptly. Alkalies, especially sodium salicylate, and intestinal antiseptics are useful. Calcium chloride in doses of five to twenty [Pg 56] grains should be tried in obstinate cases. The diet should be, for the time, of a simple character.

What systemic measures are to be prescribed in chronic and recurrent urticaria?

The cause must be sought for and treatment directed toward its removal or modification. Treatment will, therefore, depend upon indications. In obscure cases, quinine, sodium salicylate, arsenic, pilocarpine, *atropia*, potassium bromide, calcium chloride, and ichthyol are to be variously tried; general galvanization is at times useful, as is also a change of scene and climate. A proper dietary and the maintenance of free action of the bowels, preferably, as a rule, with a saline laxative, is of great importance in these chronic cases.

In acute circumscribed œdema treatment is essentially that of urticaria, the diet being given special attention.

What external applications would you advise for the relief of the subjective symptoms?

Cooling lotions of alcohol and water or vinegar and water; lotions of carbolic acid, one to three drachms to the pint; of thymol, one-fourth to one drachm to the pint of alcohol and water; of liquor carbonis detergens, one to three ounces to the pint of water, or the following:—

℞ Acidi carbolici, ... ʒj-ʒiij Acidi borici, ... ʒiv Glycerinæ, ... fʒj Alcoholis, ... f℥ij Aquæ, ... f℥xiv. M.

Alkaline baths are also useful, and may advantageously be followed by dusting-powders of starch and zinc oxide.

Urticaria Pigmentosa.

(*Synonym:* Xanthelasmoidea.)

Describe urticaria pigmentosa.

Urticaria pigmentosa is a rare disease, variously viewed as an unusual form of urticaria and as an urticaria-like eruption in which [Pg 57] there is an element of new growth in the lesions. It begins usually in infancy or early childhood and continues for months or years, and is characterized by slightly, moderately, or intensely itchy, wheal-like elevations, which are more or less persistent and leave yellowish, orange-colored, greenish or brownish stains. Exceptionally subjective symptoms are almost entirely absent. Anatomical studies show that the lesion has in some respects the structure of an ordinary wheal, with œdema and pigment deposit in the epidermal portion, and cellular infiltration made up principally of mast-cells.

Fig. 13.

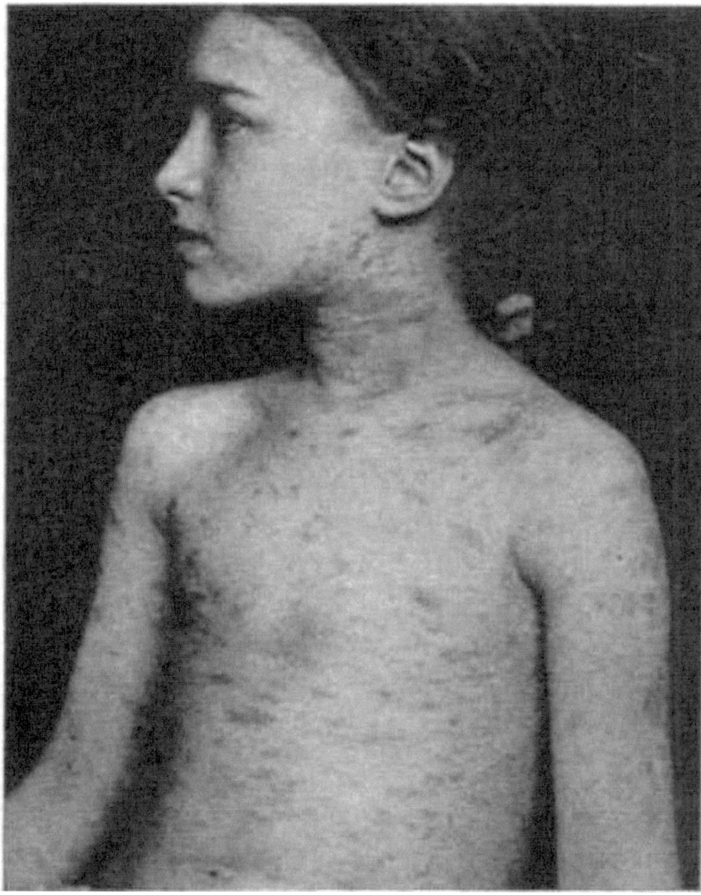

Urticaria Pigmentosa.

The nature of the disease is obscure and treatment unsatisfactory. Ordinarily as early youth or adult life is reached it spontaneously disappears. The treatment advised is usually on the same lines as that of chronic urticaria. [Pg 58]

Dermatitis.

What is implied by the term dermatitis?

Dermatitis, or inflammation of the skin, is a term employed to designate those cases of cutaneous disturbance, usually acute in character, which are due to the action of irritants.

Mention some examples of cutaneous disturbance to which this term is applied.

The dermatic inflammation due to the action of excessive heat or cold, to caustics and other chemical irritants, and to the ingestion of certain drugs.

What several varieties are commonly described?

Dermatitis traumatica, dermatitis calorica, dermatitis venenata, and dermatitis medicamentosa.

Describe dermatitis traumatica.

Under this head are included all forms of cutaneous inflammation due to traumatism. To the dermatologist the most common met with is that produced by the various animal parasites and from continued scratching; in such, if the cause has been long-continued and persistent, a variable degree of inflammatory thickening of the skin and pigmentation result, the latter not infrequently being more or less permanent. The inflammation due to tight-fitting garments, bandages, to constant pressure (as bed-sores), etc., also illustrates this class.

What is the treatment of dermatitis traumatica?

Removal of the cause, and, if necessary, the application of soothing ointments or lotions; in bed-sores, soap plaster, plain or with one to five per cent. of ichthyol.

What is dermatitis calorica?

Cutaneous inflammation, varying from a slight erythematous to a gangrenous character, produced by excessive heat (*dermatitis ambustionis, burns*) or cold (*dermatitis congelationis, frostbite*).

Give the treatment of dermatitis calorica.

In burns, if of a mild degree, the application of sodium bicarbonate, as a powder or saturated solution, is useful; in the more severe [Pg 59] grade, a two- to five-per-cent. solution will probably be found of greater advantage. Other soothing applications may also be employed. In recent years a one-per-cent. solution of picric acid has been commended for the slighter burns of limited extent. Upon the whole, there is nothing yet so generally useful and soothing in these cases as the so-called Carron oil; in some cases more valuable with 1/2 to 1 minim of carbolic acid added to each ounce.

In frostbite, seen immediately after exposure, the parts are to be brought gradually back to a normal temperature, at first by rubbing with snow or applying cold water. Subsequently, in ordinary chilblains, stimulating applications, such as oil of turpentine, balsam of Peru, tincture of iodine, ichthyol, and strongly carbolized ointments are of most benefit. If the frostbite is of a vesicular, pustular, bullous, or escharotic character, the treatment consists in the application of soothing remedies, such as are employed in other like inflammatory conditions.

What do you understand by dermatitis venenata?

All inflammatory conditions of the skin due to contact with deleterious substances such as caustic, chemical irritants, iodoform, etc., are included under this head, but the most common causes are the rhus plants—*poison ivy* (or *poison oak*) and *poison sumach* (*poison dogwood*). Mere proximity to these plants will, in some individuals, provoke cutaneous disturbance (*rhus poisoning, ivy poisoning*), although they may be handled by others with impunity.

Many other plants are also known to produce cutaneous irritation in certain subjects; among these may be mentioned the nettle, primrose, cowhage, smartweed, balm of Gilead, oleander, and rue.

The local action of iodoform (*iodoform dermatitis*) in some individuals is that of a decided irritant, bringing about a dermatitis, which often spreads much beyond the parts of application, and which in those eczematously inclined may result in a veritable and persistent eczema.

Describe the symptoms of rhus poisoning.

The symptoms appear usually soon after exposure, and consist of an inflammatory condition of the skin of an eczematous nature, [Pg 60] varying in degree from an erythematous to a bullous character, and with or without œdema and swelling. As a rule, marked itching and burning are present. The face, hands, forearms and genitalia are favorite parts, although it may in many instances involve a greater portion of the whole surface.

What is the course of rhus poisoning?

It runs an acute course, terminating in recovery in one to six weeks. In those eczematously inclined, however, it may result in a veritable and persistent form of that disease.

How would you treat rhus poisoning?

By soothing and astringent applications, such as are employed in acute eczema (*q. v.*), which are to be used freely. Among the most valuable are: a lotion of fluid extract of grindelia robusta, one to two drachms to four ounces of water; lotio nigra, either alone or followed by the oxide-of-zinc ointment; a saturated solution of boric acid, with a half to two drachms of carbolic acid to the pint; a lotion of zinc sulphate, a half to four grains to the ounce; weak alkaline lotions; cold cream, petrolatum, and oxide-of-zinc ointments.

How would you treat the dermatitis due to other deleterious substances of this class?

By applications of a soothing and protective character, similar to those used in eczema and burns.

Dermatitis Medicamentosa.

What do you understand by dermatitis medicamentosa?

Under this head are included all eruptions due to the ingestion or absorption of certain drugs.

In rare instances one dose will have such effect; commonly, however, it results only after several days' or weeks' continued administration. With some drugs such effect is the rule, with others it is exceptional, nor are all individuals equally susceptible.

How is the eruption produced in dermatitis medicamentosa?

In some instances it is probably due to the elimination of the drug through the cutaneous structures; in others, to the action of the drug upon the nervous system. The view that the drug acts as a toxin or generates some toxin or irritant material in the blood, to which the eruptive phenomena may be due, has also been advanced.

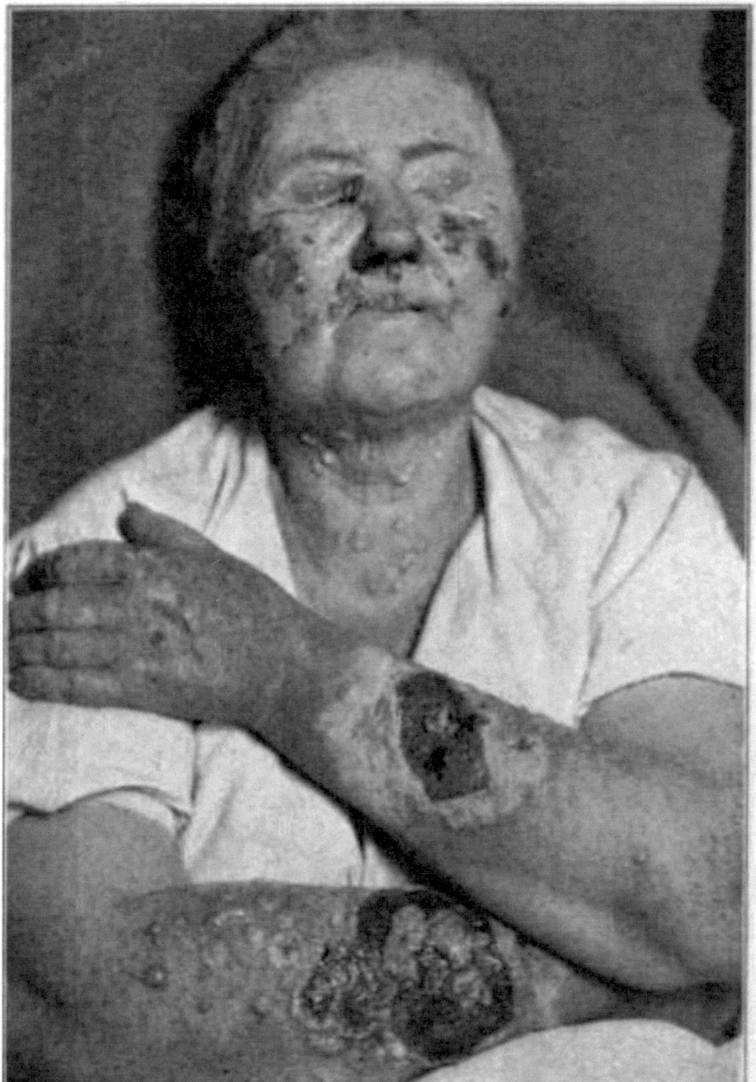

Dermatitis medicamentosa. Bullous dermatitis from iodide of potassium.

[Pg 61]

What is the character of the eruption in dermatitis medicamentosa?

It may be erythematous, papular, urticarial, vesicular, pustular or bullous, and, if the administration of the drug is continued, even gangrenous.

Name the more common drugs having such action.

Antipyrin, arsenic, atropia (or belladonna), bromides, chloral, copaiba, cubebs, digitalis, iodides, mercury, opium (or morphia), quinine, salicylic acid, stramonium, acetanilid, sulphonal, phenacetin, turpentine, many of the new coal-tar derivatives, etc.

State frequency and types of eruption due to the ingestion of antipyrin.

Not uncommon. *Erythematous*, morbilliform and erythemato-papular; itching is usually present and moderate desquamation may follow. Acetanilid, sulphonal, phenacetin, and other drugs of this class may provoke like eruptions.

Mention frequency and types of eruption due to the ingestion of arsenic.

Rare. Erythematous, erythemato-papular; exceptionally, herpetic, and pigmentary. Herpes zoster has been thought to follow its use. Keratosis of the palms and soles has also been occasionally observed, which, in rare instances, has developed into epithelioma.

Mention frequency and types of eruption due to the ingestion of atropia (or belladonna).

Not uncommon. *Erythematous* and *scarlatinoid*; usually no febrile disturbance, and desquamation seldom follows.

Give frequency and types of cutaneous disturbance following the administration of the bromides (bromine).

Common. *Pustular*, sometimes furuncular and carbuncular and superficially ulcerative. In exceptional instances papillomatous or vegetating lesions have been observed. Co-administration of arsenic or potassium bitartrate is thought to have a preventive influence in some cases. [Pg 62]

State frequency and types of cutaneous disturbance due to the administration of chloral.

Occasional. Scarlatinoid and urticarial, and exceptionally purpuric; in rare instances, if drug is continued, eruption becomes vesicular, hemorrhagic, ulcerative and even gangrenous.

State frequency and types of eruption following the administration of copaiba.

Not uncommon. *Urticarial*, erythemato-papular and *scarlatinoid*.

Mention frequency and types of eruption resulting from the ingestion of cubebs.

Uncommon. Erythematous and small papular.

Fig. 14.

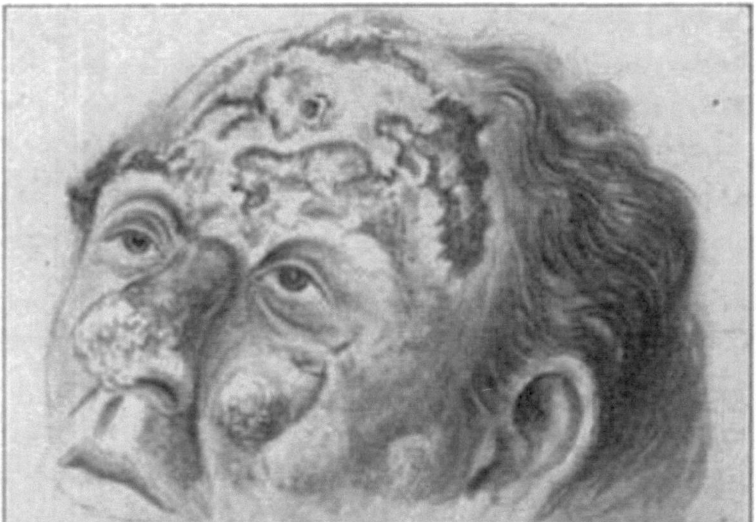

A somewhat rare form of eruption from the ingestion of iodine compounds.

(*After J.C. McGuire.*)

Mention frequency and types of eruption resulting from the administration of digitalis.

Exceptional. Scarlatinoid and papular.

State frequency and types of eruption resulting from the iodides (iodine).

Common. *Pustular*, but may be erythematous, papular, vesicular, bullous, tuberous, purpuric and hemorrhagic. Co-administration of arsenic or potassium bitartrate is thought to have a preventive influence in some cases. [Pg 63]

Give the frequency and types of eruption observed to follow the administration of mercury.

Exceptional. Erythematous and erysipelatous.

Give the frequency and types of the cutaneous disturbance following the ingestion of opium (or morphia).

Not uncommon. Erythematous and *scarlatinoid*, and sometimes urticarial.

Mention the frequency and the types of eruption following the administration of quinine.

Not infrequent. Usually *erythematous*, but may be urticarial, erythemato-papular, and even purpuric. There is, in some instances, preceding or accompanying systemic disturbance. Furfuraceous or lamellar desquamation often follows.

State frequency and types of eruption resulting from the ingestion of salicylic acid.

Not common. Erythematous and urticarial; exceptionally, vesicular, pustular, bullous, and ecchymotic.

Give frequency and type of cutaneous disturbance due to the administration of stramonium.

Not common. Erythematous.

State frequency and types of eruption resulting from the administration of turpentine.

Not uncommon. *Erythematous,* and small-papular; exceptionally vesicular.

X-Ray Dermatitis.

What several grades of x-ray dermatitis (x-ray burns, Rontgen-ray burns) are observed?

Three grades are usually described: erythema, superficial vesication, and necrosis. The first and second may come on shortly—a few hours to several days—after exposure; occasionally later. The third grade may present also in the first several days, but in many cases one to several weeks may elapse before it appears; it is quite commonly preceded by erythema and vesication. The necrosis may be superficial or deep, and quite usually results in a persistent ulcer covered by a leathery coating; it is usually painful. [Pg 64]

Give the prognosis and treatment of x-ray dermatitis.

The first grade—the erythematous—usually disappears in one to ten days; the second grade requires one to several weeks, and may be quite sore and tender; the severe or necrotic burns are persistent, sometimes lasting for months and several years, with little tendency to spontaneous disappearance, and rebellious to treatment.

Fig. 15.

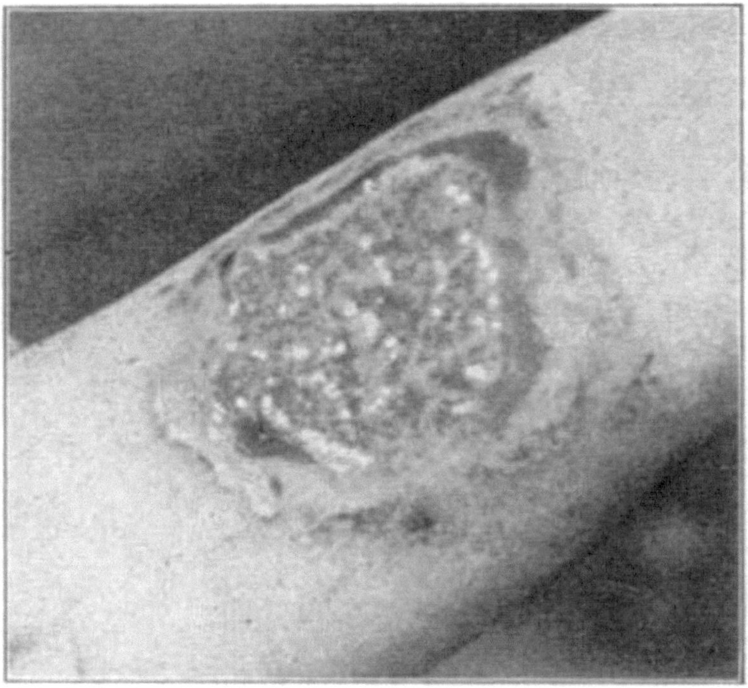

x-ray burn

Treatment of the milder types is that of erythema (*q. v.*); the necrotic type occasionally demands thorough curetting and skin-grafting before it will heal.

Dermatitis Factitia.

(*Synonym:* Feigned Eruptions.)

What do you understand by feigned eruptions?

Feigned, or artificial, eruptions, occasionally met with in hysterical females and in others, are produced, for the purpose of exciting sympathy or of deception, by the action of friction, cantharides, acids or [Pg 65] strong alkalies; the cutaneous disturbance may, therefore, be erythematous, vesicular, bullous, or gangrenous. It is usually limited in extent, and, as a rule, seen only on parts easily reached by the hands.

Fig. 16.

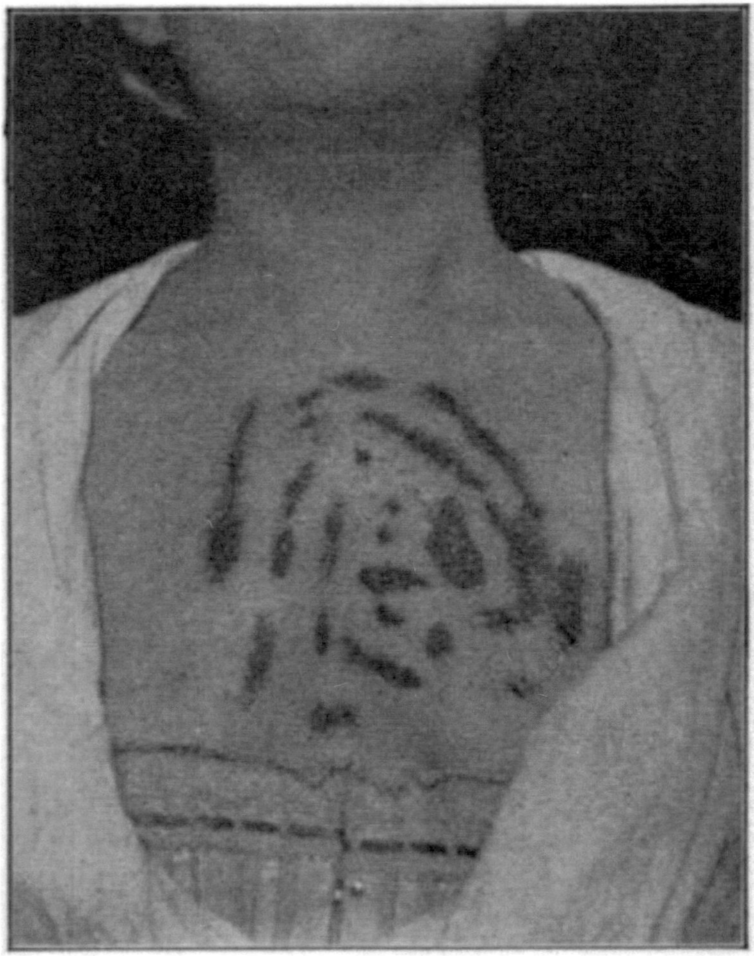

Dermatitis Factitia—note the unusually uniform and regular character and arrangement of the lesions.

Dermatitis Gangrænosa.

Dermatitis Gangrænosa.

What do you understand by dermatitis gangrænosa?

Dermatitis gangrænosa (*erythema gangrænosum, Raynaud's disease, spontaneous gangrene*) is an exceedingly rare affection, characterized by the formation of gangrenous spots and patches. It [Pg 66] may be idiopathic or symptomatic. Some of these cases, especially in hysterical subjects, belong under the "feigned eruptions," being self-produced.

As an idiopathic disease, it begins as erythematous, dark-red spots—usually preceded and accompanied by mild or grave systemic disturbance—which gradually pass into gangrene and sloughing; the eventual termination may be fatal, or recovery may take place. As a symptomatic disease, it is occasionally met with in diabetes and in grave cerebral and spinal affections.

In Raynaud's disease (symmetric gangrene) the parts affected are the extremities, such as fingers and toes, the ears and nose, only occasionally other parts. The first symptoms observed are coldness and paleness of the part; followed sooner or later by congestion of a dark red, livid, or bluish color, with sometimes swelling, and tenderness and shooting pains. The termination is usually in gangrene of a dry character, with, in some instances, vesicles and blebs along the edges; in other cases the parts become atrophied, withered, and indurated.

Treatment is based upon general principles.

Erysipelas.

What is erysipelas?

Erysipelas is an acute specific inflammation of the skin and subcutaneous tissue, commonly of the face, characterized by shining redness, swelling, œdema, heat, and a tendency in some cases to vesicle- and bleb-formation, and accompanied by more or less febrile disturbance.

Describe the symptoms and course of erysipelas.

A decided rigor or a feeling of chilliness followed by febrile action usually ushers in the cutaneous disturbance. The skin at a certain point or part, commonly where there is a lesion of continuity, becomes bright red and swollen; this spreads by peripheral extension, and in the course of several hours involves a portion or the whole region. The parts are shining red, swollen, of an elevated temperature, and sharply defined against the sound skin. After several days or a week, during which time there is usually continued mild or severe febrile action, the process begins to subside, and is followed by epidermic desquamation. [Pg 67]

In some cases vesicles and blebs may be present; in other cases the disease seriously involves the deeper parts, and is accompanied by grave constitutional symptoms. In exceptional instances sloughing takes place.

A mild, transitory, limited, and often recurrent erysipelatous condition of the outlet and immediate neighborhood of one or both nostrils is met with, taking its origin from an inflammation of the hair-follicles just inside the margin of the nose; constitutional symptoms are usually wanting. Somewhat similar, doubtless, is the erysipelatous inflammation (*erysipeloid*) observed on the fingers and hands of butchers, etc., starting from a wound, apparently as a result of infection from putrid meat or fish.

What is erysipelas migrans (or erysipelas ambulans)?

A variety of erysipelas which, after a few hours or days, disappears at one region and appears at another, and so continues for one or several weeks.

What is the cause of erysipelas?

The disease is due to a specific streptococcus—the streptococcus of Fehleisen. Depression of the vital forces and local abrasions are predisposing factors.

State the diagnostic points.

The character of the onset, the shining redness and swelling, the sharply-defined border, and the accompanying febrile disturbance.

What is the prognosis in erysipelas?

In most instances the disease runs a favorable course, terminating in recovery in one to three weeks. Exceptionally, in severe cases, a fatal termination ensues.

What is the treatment of erysipelas?

Internally, a purge, followed by the tincture of the chloride of iron and quinia, and stimulants if needed. *Locally*, one to three per cent. carbolic-acid lotion or ointment, a saturated solution of boric acid, or a ten- to twenty-per-cent. aqueous solution or ointment of ichthyol may be employed.

In some cases the spread of the disease is apparently controlled by painting the bordering healthy skin with a ring of tincture of iodine or strong solution of nitrate of silver. [Pg 68]

Phlegmona Diffusa.

What do you understand by phlegmona diffusa?

Phlegmona diffusa is a more or less extensive inflammation of the cutaneous and subcutaneous tissues presenting symptoms partaking of the nature of both deep erysipelas and flat carbuncles, and usually attended with varying constitutional disturbance. Suppuration at several points takes place, and sloughing may ensue. Recovery usually finally results, but a fatal issue is possible.

Treatment is based upon general principles.

Furunculus.

(*Synonyms:* Furuncle; Boil.)

Define furunculus.

Furunculus, or boil, is an acute, deep-seated, inflammatory, circumscribed, rounded or more or less acuminated, firm, painful formation, usually terminating in central suppuration.

Describe the symptoms and course.

A boil begins as a small, rounded or imperfectly defined reddish spot, or as a small, superficial pustule; it increases in size, and when well advanced appears as a pea or cherry-sized, circumscribed, reddish elevation, with more or less surrounding hyperæmia and swelling; it is painful and tender, and ends, in the course of several days or a week, in the formation of a central slough or "*core*," which finally involves the central overlying skin (*pointing*). One or several may be present, gradually maturing and disappearing. Insignificant scarring may remain.

In some cases sympathetic constitutional disturbance is noticed.

What is a blind boil?

A sluggish boil exhibiting little, if any, tendency to point or break.

What is furunculosis?

Furunculosis is that condition in which boils, singly or in crops, continue to appear, irregularly, for weeks or months. [Pg 69]

State the etiology of furuncle.

A depraved state of the general health is often to be considered as a predisposing factor. Persistent furunculosis is not infrequent in diabetes mellitus. The immediate exciting cause is the entrance into the follicle of a microbe, the staphylococcus pyogenes aureus. It is not improbable, however, that boils may also be due to other pus-producing organisms.

Workmen in paraffin oils or other petroleum products often present numerous furuncles and cutaneous abscesses. Conditions favoring a persistent miliaria have also a causative influence, especially observed in infants and young children. In these latter, especially among the poorer classes, sluggish boils or subcutaneous abscesses about the scalp in hot weather, are not at all infrequent.

What is the pathology of furuncle?

A boil is an inflammatory formation having its starting point in a sebaceous-gland, sweat-gland, or hair-follicle. The core, or central slough, is composed of pus and of the tissue of the gland in which it had its origin.

How would you distinguish a boil from a carbuncle?

A boil is comparatively small, rounded or acuminate, and has but one point of suppuration; a carbuncle is large, flattened, intensely painful, often with grave systemic disturbance, and has, moreover, several centres of suppuration.

State the prognosis.

When occurring in crops (furunculosis) the affection is often rebellious; recovery, however, finally resulting.

What is the method of treatment of furunculus?

If there be but one lesion, with no tendency to the appearance of others, local treatment alone is usually employed. If, however, several or more are present, or if there is a tendency to successive development, both constitutional and local measures are demanded.

Name the internal remedies employed.

Such nutrients and tonics as cod-liver oil, malt, quinine, strychnia, iron and arsenic; in some instances calx sulphurata, one-tenth- to [Pg 70] one-fourth-grain doses every three or four hours has been thought to be of service. Brewers' yeast has been recently again brought forward as a remedy of value.

What is the external treatment?

Local treatment consists in the beginning, with the hope of aborting the lesion, of the application of carbolic acid to the central portion, or the use of a twenty-five-per-cent. ointment of ichthyol applied as a plaster:—

℞ Ichthyol, ... ʒj Emp. plumbi, ... ʒij Emp. resinæ, ... ʒj.
M.

Or the injection of a five-per-cent. solution of carbolic acid into the apex of the boil may be tried if the formation is more advanced. If suppuration is fully established, evacuation of the contents, followed by antiseptic applications, constitutes the best method.

A saturated solution of boric acid or a lotion of corrosive sublimate (one to three grains to the ounce) applied to the immediate neighborhood of the boil or boils tends to prevent the formation of new lesions. Frequent washing of the parts with soap and water or tincture of green soap and water is also a preventive measure of value. In repeatedly infected areas, mild exposures to *x*-rays, at intervals of a few days, will often prove of curative value.

Carbunculus.

(*Synonyms:* Anthrax; Carbuncle.)

What is carbuncle?

A carbuncle is an acute, usually egg to palm-sized, circumscribed, phlegmonous inflammation of the skin and subcutaneous structures, terminating in a slough.

At what age and upon what parts is carbuncle usually observed?

In middle and advanced life, and more commonly in men.

It is seen most frequently at the nape of the neck and upon the upper part of the back. [Pg 71]

What are the symptoms and course of carbuncle?

There is rarely more than one lesion present. It begins, usually with preceding and accompanying malaise, chilliness and febrile disturbance, as a firm, flat, inflammatory infiltration in the deeper skin and subcutaneous tissue, spreading laterally and finally involving an area of one to several inches in diameter. The infiltration and swelling increase, the skin becomes of dark red color, and sooner or later, usually at the end of ten days or two weeks, softening and suppuration begin to take place, the skin finally giving away at several points, through which sanious pus exudes; the whole mass finally sloughs away either in portions or in its entirety, resulting in a deep ulcer, which slowly heals and leaves a permanent cicatrix.

In some cases, especially in old people, constitutional disturbance of a grave character is noted, septicæmia is developed, and a fatal result may ensue.

What is the cause of carbuncle?

The same causes are considered to be operative in carbunculus as in furuncle; general debility and depression, from whatever cause, predisposing to its formation, and the introduction of a microbe, probably the same as in furunculus, being at present looked upon as the exciting factor.

What is the pathology?

The inflammation starts simultaneously from numerous points, from the hair-follicles, sweat-glands or sebaceous glands. The inflammatory centres break down, and the pus finds its way to the surface; finally the process ends in gangrene of the whole area.

How would you distinguish carbuncle from a boil?

By its flat character, greater size, and multiple points of suppuration.

What is the prognosis of carbuncle?

Occurring in those greatly debilitated or in late life, and in those cases in which two or more lesions exist, or when seated about the head, the prognosis is always to be guarded, as a fatal result is not uncommon. In fact, in every instance the disease is to be considered of possible serious import. [Pg 72]

What constitutional treatment is usually employed in carbuncle?

A full nutritious diet, the use of such remedies as iron, quinia, nux vomica, with malt and stimulants, if indicated. Calx sulphurata, one-tenth to one-fourth grain every two or three hours, appears, in some instances, to have a beneficial effect. If the pain is severe, morphia or chloral should be given.

What external measures are employed?

In the early part of the formation, injection of a five or ten per cent. carbolic acid solution, or covering the whole area with a twenty-five per cent. ichthyol ointment, may be employed. When it has broken down the pus may be drawn out with a cupping-glass, and carbolized glycerine or carbolized water introduced into each opening, and the ichthyol ointment superimposed. If the whole part has sloughed, it should be removed as rapidly as possible, and antiseptic dressings used. Or, if its progress is slow, and grave systemic disturbance be present, the whole part may be incised and curetted, and then treated antiseptically. Mild exposure to the *x*-rays is also to be commended.

Pustula Maligna.

(*Synonyms:* Anthrax; Malignant Pustule.)

What is malignant pustule?

Malignant pustule is a furuncle- or carbuncle-like lesion resulting from inoculation of the virus generated in animals suffering from splenic fever, or "charbon," and is accompanied by constitutional symptoms of more or less gravity. A fatal termination is not unusual.

What is the cause of pustula maligna?

The disease is due to the presence of the bacillus anthracis.

What is the treatment of malignant pustule?

Early excision or destruction with caustic potash, with subsequent antiseptic dressings; and internally the free use of stimulants and tonics. [Pg 73]

Post-mortem Pustule.

(*Synonym:* Dissection Wound.)

Describe post-mortem pustule.

Post-mortem pustule develops at the point of inoculation, beginning as an itchy red spot, becoming vesico-pustular, and later pustular, with usually a broad inflammatory base, and accompanied with more or less pain and redness and not infrequently lymphangitis, erysipelatous swelling, and slight or severe sympathetic constitutional disturbance.

What is the treatment of post-mortem pustule?

Treatment consists in opening the pustule and thorough cauterization, and the subsequent use of antiseptic applications or dressings. *Internally* quinia and stimulants if indicated.

Frambœsia.

(*Synonyms:* Yaws; Pian.)

Describe frambœsia.

Frambœsia is an endemic, contagious disease met with in tropical countries, characterized by the appearance of variously-sized papules, tubercles, and tumors, which, when developed, resemble currants and small raspberries, and finally break down and ulcerate. It is accompanied by constitutional symptoms of variable severity.

Hygienic measures, good food, tonics, and antiseptic and stimulating applications are curative.

Verruga Peruana.

(*Synonyms:* Peruvian Warts; Carrion's Disease; Oroya Fever.)

Describe verruga peruana.

A specific inoculable affection endemic in some valleys of the Western Andes, in Peru, and characterized by a prodromal febrile period and subsequent outbreak of peculiar pin-head- to pea-sized, or larger, bright reddish, rounded, wart-like elevations. The prodromal symptoms, of an irregular malarial or typhoid type, with associated rheumatic and muscular pains, may last for weeks or several months, [Pg 74] usually abating when eruption presents. The lesions may be crowded together in great bunches. The face and limbs are favorite localities. The disease is inoculable and thought to be due to a bacillus.

The fatality varies between 10 and 20 per cent. Tonics and stimulants are prescribed.

Equinia.

(*Synonyms:* Farcy; Glanders.)

What is equinia, or glanders?

A rare contagious specific disease of a malignant type, derived from the horse, and characterized by grave constitutional symptoms, inflammation of the nasal and respiratory passages, and a deep-seated papulo-pustular, or tubercular, nodular (*farcy buds*), ulcerative eruption. A fatal issue is not uncommon. It is due to a micro-organism.

Treatment, both local and constitutional, is based upon general principles.

Miliaria.

(*Synonyms:* Prickly Heat; Heat Rash; Lichen Tropicus; Red Gum; Strophulus.)

What do you understand by miliaria?

An acute mildly inflammatory disorder of the sweat-glands, characterized by the appearance of minute, discrete but closely crowded papules, vesico-papules, and vesicles.

Describe the symptoms of miliaria.

The eruption, consisting of pin-point to millet-seed-sized papules, vesico-papules, vesicles, or a mixture of these lesions, discrete but usually numerous and closely crowded, appears suddenly, occurring upon a limited portion of the surface, or, as commonly observed, involving a greater part or the whole integument. The trunk is a favorite locality. The papular lesions are pinkish or reddish, and the vesicles whitish or yellowish, surrounded by inflammatory areola, thus giving the whole eruption a bright red appearance—*miliaria rubra*. Later, the areolæ fade, the transparent contents of the vesicles become somewhat opaque and yellowish-white, and the [Pg 75] eruption has a whitish or yellowish cast—*miliaria alba*. In long-continued cases, especially in children, boils and cutaneous abscesses sometimes develop; and it may also develop into a true eczema.

Itching, or a feeling of burning, slight or intense, is usually present.

What is the course of the eruption?

The vesicles show no disposition to rupture, but dry up in a few days or a week, disappearing by absorption and with slight subsequent desquamation; the papular lesions gradually fade away, and the affection, if the exciting cause has ceased to act, terminates.

What is the cause of miliaria?

Excessive heat. Debilitated individuals, especially children, are more prone to an attack. Being too warmly clad is often causative.

What is the nature of the disease?

The affection is considered to be due to sweat-obstruction, with mild inflammatory symptoms as a cause or consequence, congestion and exudation taking place about the ducts, giving rise to papules or vesicles, according to the intensity of the process.

How would you distinguish miliaria from papular and vesicular eczema, and from sudamen?

The papules of eczema are larger, more elevated, firmer, slower in their evolution, of longer duration, and are markedly itchy.

The vesicles of eczema are usually larger, tend to become confluent, and also to rupture and become crusted; there is marked itchiness, and the inflammatory action is usually severe and persistent.

In sudamen there is absence of inflammatory symptoms.

What is the prognosis of miliaria?

The affection, under favorable circumstances, disappears in a few days or weeks. If the cause persists, as for instance, in infants or young children too warmly clad, it may result in eczema.

What is the treatment of miliaria?

Removal of the cause, and in debilitated subjects the administration of tonics; together with the application of cooling and astringent lotions, as the following:— [Pg 76]

> ℞ Aeidi carbolici, ... ʒss-ʒj Acidi borici,
> .... ʒiv Glycerinæ, ... fʒj
> Alcoholis, ... f℥ij Aquæ,
> .... ℥xiv. M.

This is sometimes more efficient if zinc oxide, six to eight drachms, is added.

Lotions of alcohol and water or vinegar and water, and also the various lotions used in acute eczema, are often employed with relief.

Dusting-powders of starch, boric acid, lycopodium, talc, and zinc oxide are also valuable; the following combination is satisfactory:—

℞ Pulv. acidi borici, Pulv. talci veneti, Pulv. zinci oxidi, Pulv. amyli, ...āā......... ʒij. M.

Probably the best plan is to use a lotion and a dusting-powder conjointly; dabbing on the wash freely, allowing it to dry, and then dusting over with the powder.

Pompholyx.

(*Synonyms:* Dysidrosis; Cheiro-pompholyx.)

What is pompholyx?

Pompholyx is a rare disease of the skin of a vesicular and bullous character, and limited to the hands and feet.

Describe the symptoms of pompholyx.

In most instances the hands only are affected. It begins usually with a feeling of burning, tingling or tenderness of the parts, followed rapidly by the appearance of deeply-seated vesicles, especially between the fingers and on the palmar aspect. These beginning lesions look not unlike sago grains imbedded in the skin. In some instances the disease does not extend beyond this stage, the vesicles disappearing after a few days or weeks by absorption, and usually [Pg 77] without desquamation. Ordinarily, however, the lesions increase in size, new ones arise, become confluent, and blebs result, the skin in places appearing as if undermined with serous exudation. The parts are commonly inflamed to a slight or marked degree. The skin comes off in flakes, new lesions may appear for several days or two or three weeks, and the process then declines, recovery gradually taking place.

There are no constitutional symptoms, although it is usually noticed that the general health is below par.

What is the character of the subjective symptoms in pompholyx?

The subjective symptoms consist of a feeling of tension, burning and tenderness, and sometimes itching. Not infrequently, also there is neuralgic pain.

What is the cause of pompholyx?

The eruption is thought to be due to a depressed state of the nervous system. It is more common in women, and is met with chiefly in adult and middle life.

What is the pathology?

Opinion is divided; some considering it a disease of the sweat-glands and others an inflammatory disease independent of these structures.

State the diagnostic features of pompholyx.

The distribution and the peculiar characters and course of the eruption.

It is to be differentiated from eczema.

What is the prognosis?

For the immediate attack, favorable, recovery taking place in several weeks or a few months. Recurrences at irregular intervals are not uncommon.

What is the treatment of pompholyx?

The general health is to be looked after, and the patient placed under good hygienic conditions. Remedies of a tonic nature, directed especially toward improving the state of the nervous system, are to be prescribed. *Locally*, soothing and anodyne applications, [Pg 78] such as lead-water and laudanum, boric-acid lotion, oxide-of-zinc, boric-acid and diachylon ointments, are most suitable; or the parts may be enveloped with the following:—

> ℞ Pulv. ac. salicylici, ... gr. x Pulv. ac. borici, Pulv. amyli, ...āā................. ʒij Petrolati, ... ʒiv. M.

In fact, the external treatment is similar to that employed in acute eczema.

Herpes Simplex.

(*Synonym:* Fever Blisters.)

What is herpes simplex?

An acute inflammatory disease, characterized by the formation of pin-head to pea-sized vesicles, arranged in groups, and occurring for the most part about the face and genitalia.

Describe the symptoms of herpes simplex.

In severe cases, malaise and pyrexia may precede the eruption, but usually it appears without any precursory or constitutional symptoms. A feeling of heat and burning in the parts is often complained of. The vesicles, which are commonly pin-head in size, are usually upon a hyperæmic or inflammatory base, and tend to occur in groups or clusters. Their contents are usually clear, subsequently becoming more or less milky or puriform. There is no tendency to spontaneous rupture, but should they be broken a superficial excoriation results. In a short time they dry to crusts which soon fall off, leaving no permanent trace.

Is the eruption in herpes simplex abundant?

No. As a rule not more than one or two clusters or groups are observed.

Upon what parts does the eruption occur?

Usually about the face (*herpes facialis*), and most frequently about the lips (*herpes labialis*); on the genitalia (*herpes progenitalis*), the [Pg 79] lesions are commonly found on the prepuce (*herpes præputialis*) in the male, and on the labia minora and labia majora in the female.

State the causes of herpes simplex.

Herpes facialis is often observed in association with colds and febrile and lung diseases. Malaria, digestive disturbance, and nervous disorders are not infrequently predisposing factors. Herpes progenitalis is said to occur more frequently in those who have previously had some venereal disease, especially gonorrhœa, but this is questionable. It is probably often purely neurotic.

What are the diagnostic points?

The appearance of one or several vesicular groups or clusters about the face, and especially about the lips, is usually sufficiently characteristic. The same holds true ordinarily when the eruption is seen on the prepuce or other parts of the genitalia; it is only when the vesicles become rubbed or abraded and irritated that it might be mistaken for a venereal sore, but the history, course and duration will usually serve to differentiate.

Give the prognosis.

The eruption will usually disappear in several days or one or two weeks without treatment. Remedial applications, however, exert a favorable influence. Herpes progenitalis exhibits a strong disposition to recurrence.

What is the treatment of herpes facialis?

Anointing the parts with camphorated cold cream, with spirits of camphor or similar evaporating and stimulating applications will at times afford relief to the burning, and shorten the course.

What is the treatment of herpes progenitalis?

In herpes about the genitalia cleanliness is of first importance. A saturated solution of boric acid, a dusting-powder of calomel or oxide of zinc, and the following lotion, containing calamine and oxide of zinc, are valuable:—

℞ Zinci oxidi, Calaminæ, ...āā......................... gr. v Glycerinæ, Alcoholis, ...āā......................... ♏vj Aquæ, ... ℥j M.

[Pg 80] In obstinate recurrent cases, frequent applications of a mild galvanic current will have a favorable influence.

Hydroa Vacciniforme.

(*Synonyms:* Recurrent Summer Eruption; Hydroa Puerorum; Hydroa Aestivale.)

Describe hydroa vacciniforme.

It is a rare vesicular disease usually seen in boys (only two or three exceptions), occurring upon uncovered parts, especially the nose, cheeks, and ears. The lesions begin as red spots, discrete or in groups, rapidly exhibit vesiculation, and later umbilication; the contents become milky, dry to crusts, which fall off and leave small pit-like scars. Fresh outbreaks may take place almost continuously, and the process go on indefinitely, at least up to youth or manhood, when the tendency subsides. Its activity is usually limited to the warm season. Arthritic symptoms and general disturbance are sometimes noted in severe cases.

It is doubtless a vasomotor neurosis. Exposure to sun and wind is an important, if not essential, etiological factor. Primarily the lesion begins in the rete middle layers, and is purely vesicular in character; later, necrosis of the rete and extending deep in the corium is observed.

Treatment so far has only been palliative, consisting of the applications employed in similar conditions. Constitutional medication is based upon general principles. The patient should avoid exposure to the sun, strong wind and excessive artificial heat.

Epidermolysis Bullosa.

Describe epidermolysis bullosa.

This is a rare, usually hereditary, disease or condition, characterized by the formation of vesicles and blebs on any part subjected to slight rubbing or irritation. No scarring is left, and no pigmentation noted. The predisposition to these lesions persists indefinitely. The general health is not involved. The nature of the disease is obscure.

Treatment has no influence in modifying or lessening this tendency. The vulnerable parts should so far as possible be protected from knocks and undue friction. [Pg 81]

Dermatitis Repens.

What do you understand by dermatitis repens?

It is a rare spreading dermatitis starting from an injury, extending by a serous undermining of the epidermis, and usually occurring upon the upper extremities.

It usually begins shortly after an injury, and, as a rule, presents itself by redness and serous exudation. The overlying epidermis breaks, and the area of disease gradually progresses by an extension of the serous undermining process, the denuded part looking red and raw, with usually an oozing surface. As the disease spreads the oldest part becomes dry and heals, the new epidermal covering being thin and atrophic in appearance. Its most usual beginning is on some part of the hand, and from here it may spread up the arm and involve considerable area.

The injury from which it starts may be extremely insignificant, apparently affording an opening for the introduction of the causative factor, doubtless parasitic. Beyond a feeling of soreness there seem to be no special subjective symptoms.

Give the prognosis and treatment.

The malady shows but little tendency to spontaneous cure. The frequent or constant application of a mild antiseptic lotion, such as boric acid and resorcin, or of a mild parasiticide ointment will generally bring the disease gradually to an end.

Herpes Zoster.

(*Synonyms:* Zoster; Zona; Shingles.)

Give a definition of herpes zoster.

Herpes zoster is an acute, self-limited, inflammatory disease, characterized by groups of vesicles upon inflammatory bases, situated over or along a nerve tract.

Upon what parts of the body may the eruption appear?

It may appear upon any part, following the course of a nerve; it is therefore always limited in extent, and confined to one side of the body. It is probably most common about the intercostal, lumbar and supra-orbital regions. In rare instances the eruption has been observed to be bilateral. [Pg 82]

Are there any subjective or constitutional symptoms?

Yes; there is, as a rule, neuralgic pain preceding, during and following the eruption; and in some cases, also, there may be in the beginning mild febrile disturbance. There is also a variable degree of tenderness and pain.

What are the characters of the eruption?

Several or more hyperæmic or inflammatory patches over a nerve course appear, upon which are seated vesico-papules irregularly grouped; these vesico-papules become distinct vesicles, of size from a pin-head to a pea, and soon dry and give rise to thin, yellowish or brownish crusts, which drop off, leaving in most instances no permanent trace, in others more or less scarring. In some cases the lesions may become pustular and, on the other hand, the eruption may be abortive, stopping short of full vesiculation.

What is known in regard to the nature of the disease?

An inflamed and irritable state of the spinal ganglia, nerve tract, or peripheral branches is directly responsible for the eruption, and this state may be due to atmospheric changes, cold, nerve-injuries and similar influences. The view has also been advanced that the disease is of specific and infectious character.

Give the chief diagnostic features of herpes zoster.

The prodromic neuralgic pain, the appearance of grouped vesicles upon inflammatory bases following the course of a nerve tract, and the limitation of the eruption to one side of the body.

What is the prognosis?

Favorable; the symptoms usually disappearing in two to four weeks. In some instances, however, the neuralgic pains may be persistent, and in zoster of the supra-orbital region the eye may suffer permanent damage.

How would you treat herpes zoster?

Constitutional treatment, usually tonic in character, is to be based upon general principles; moderate doses of quinia, with one-sixth grain of zinc phosphide, four or five times daily, appear in some cases to have a special value. The accompanying neuralgic pain may be so intense as to require anodynes.

Local treatment should be of a soothing and protective [Pg 83] character. A dusting-powder of oxide of zinc and starch (to the ounce of which twenty to thirty grains of camphor may be added) proves useful; and over this, in order that the parts be further protected, a bandage or a layer of cotton batting. Oxide-of-zinc ointment, and in those cases in which there is much pain, ointments containing powdered opium or belladonna, or orthoform, may be used. A mild galvanic current applied daily to the parts is often of great advantage, both in its influence upon the course of the eruption and upon the neuralgic pain. The plan, so often advised, of painting the parts with flexible collodion is not to be commended.

Dermatitis Herpetiformis.

(*Synonyms:* Hydroa Herpetiforme (Tilbury Fox); Herpes Gestationis (Bulkley); Pemphigus Prurigiuosus; Duhring's Disease.)

Give a definition of dermatitis herpetiformis.

Dermatitis herpetiformis is a somewhat rare inflammatory disease, characterized by an eruption of an erythematous, papular, vesicular, pustular, bullous or mixed type, with a decided disposition toward grouping, accompanied by itching and burning sensations, with, as a rule, more or less consequent pigmentation, and pursuing usually a chronic course with remissions.

Describe the erythematous type of dermatitis herpetiformis.

The character of the eruption in the erythematous type resembles closely that of erythema multiforme and of urticaria, especially the former. The efflorescences usually make their appearance in crops, and are more or less persistent; fading sooner or later, however, and giving place to new outbreaks. Vesicles are often intermingled, developing from erythematous and erythemato-papular lesions or arising from apparently normal skin.

It may continue in the same type, or change to the vesicular, bullous or other variety.

Describe the papular type of dermatitis herpetiformis.

This is rarely seen as consisting purely of papular lesions, but is commonly associated with the erythematous and vesicular varieties. In a measure it resembles the papular manifestations of erythema multiforme, with a distinct disposition toward group formation. The [Pg 84] papules tend, sooner or later, to develop into vesicles, new papular outbreaks occurring from time to time; or the whole eruption changes to the vesicular or other type of the disease. It is not a common type.

Describe the vesicular type of dermatitis herpetiformis.

This is the common clinical type of the disease, and is characterized by pin-head to pea-sized, rounded or irregularly-shaped, distended or flattened and stellate vesicles, occurring, for the most part, in irregular and segmental groups of three or more lesions, seated either upon apparently normal integument or upon hyperæmic or inflammatory skin. They exhibit no tendency to spontaneous rupture, but after remaining a shorter or longer time, are broken or disappear by absorption. The lesions tend to appear in crops. It may, as it not infrequently does, continue in the same type, or it may become more or less erythematous or bullous in character. In not a few instances pustules, few or in numbers, are at times intermingled.

Describe the pustular type of dermatitis herpetiformis.

This is rare. It is similar in its clinical characters to the vesicular type, except that the lesions are pustular. It is met with, as a rule, in association with the vesicular and bullous varieties of the disease.

Describe the bullous type of dermatitis herpetiformis.

The bullous expression of the disease is usually of a markedly inflammatory nature, often innumerable blebs, small and large, appearing almost continuously, and in some instances involving the greater part of the surface. The lesions arise from erythematous skin, from preëxisting vesicles or vesicular groups, or from apparently normal integument. There is a marked disposition to appear in clusters. A change of type to the erythematous or vesicular varieties is not unusual.

Describe the mixed type of dermatitis herpetiformis.

In this type the eruption is made up of erythematous patches, vesicles, bullæ, and often with pustules intermingled, appearing irregularly or in crops, and with a tendency to patch or group formation.

Describe the characters of the vesicles, pustules and blebs.

As a rule, these several lesions, especially the vesicles and blebs, are somewhat peculiar: they are usually of a strikingly irregular [Pg 85] outline, oblong, stellate, quadrate, and when drying are apt to have a puckered appearance. They are herpetic in that they show little disposition to spontaneous rupture, occur in groups, and are usually seated upon erythematous or inflammatory skin—in some respects similar to the groups of simple herpes and herpes zoster.

What is to be said in regard to the subjective symptoms?

The subjective symptoms are usually the most troublesome feature of the disease, consisting of intense and persistent itching and a feeling of heat and burning.

Are there any constitutional symptoms in dermatitis herpetiformis?

As a rule, not, excepting the distress and depression necessarily consequent upon the intense itchiness and loss of sleep. In the pustular and bullous varieties there may be mild or grave systemic symptoms, but even in these types the constitutional involvement is, in most instances, slight in comparison to the intensity of the cutaneous disturbance.

What is the course of dermatitis herpetiformis?

Extremely chronic, in most instances lasting, with remissions, indefinitely. The skin is rarely entirely free. From time to time the type of the disease may undergo change. From the continued irritation and scratching more or less pigmentation results.

What is to be said in regard to the etiology?

The disease is in many instances essentially neurotic, and in exceptional instances septicæmic. Pregnancy and the parturient state are factors in some instances (so-called herpes gestationis). It is possible in some instances that the eruption may be an expression of a mild toxemia of gastro-intestinal origin. In some cases no cause can be assigned. In the majority of patients the general health, considering the violence of the eruptive phenomena, remains comparatively undisturbed.

Nervous shock and mental worry are factors in some cases. Polyuria, with sugar in the urine, has occasionally been noted. Eosinophile cells have been found both in the vesicles and the blood. In some instances—exceptionally, it is true—the disease has appeared shortly after vaccination.

Mention the diagnostic features of dermatitis herpetiformis.

The multiformity of the eruption, the characters of the lesions, [Pg 86] the disposition to grouping, the absence of tendency to form solid sheets of eruption (as in eczema), the intense itching, history, chronicity and course. In doubtful cases, an observation of several weeks will always suffice to distinguish it from eczema, erythema multiforme, herpes iris and pemphigus, diseases to which it at times bears strong resemblance.

Give the prognosis of dermatitis herpetiformis.

An opinion as to the outcome of the disease should be guarded. It is exceedingly rebellious to treatment, and relapses are the rule. Exceptionally the bullous and pustular varieties prove eventually fatal. The erythematous and vesicular varieties are the most favorable.

State the treatment to be advised.

There are no special remedies. Constitutional treatment must be conducted upon general principles. A free action of the bowels is to be maintained. In occasional instances arsenic in progressive doses seems of value. Externally protective and antipruritic applications, such as are employed in the treatment of eczema and pemphigus, are to be employed:—

℞ Ac. carbolici, ... ʒj-ʒij Thymol,
.... gr. xvj. Glycerinæ,
.... ℥ss-℥j Alcoholis, ...
f℥ij Aquæ, q.s., ...ad........................... Oj. M.

Other valuable applications are: lotions of carbolic acid, of liquor carbonis detergens, of boric acid; alkaline baths, mild sulphur ointment and carbolized oxide-of-zinc ointment, and dusting-powders of starch, zinc oxide, talc and boric acid. A two- to ten-per-cent. ichthyol lotion or ointment is sometimes of advantage; thiol employed in the same manner has also been commended.

Psoriasis.

Give a definition of psoriasis.

Psoriasis is a chronic, inflammatory disease, characterized by dry, reddish, variously-sized, rounded, sharply-defined, more or less infiltrated, scaly patches.

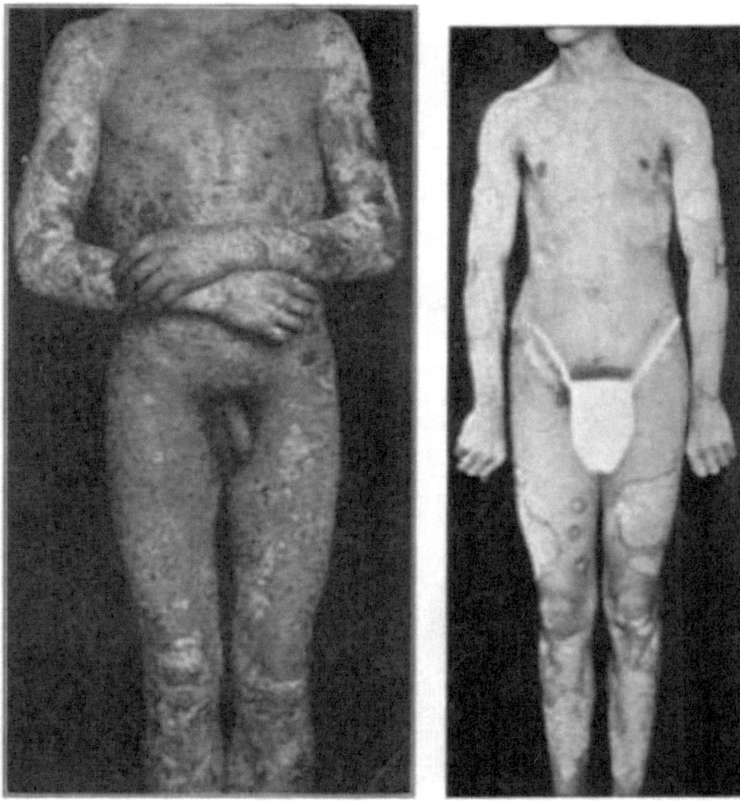

Psoriasis.

[Pg 87]

At what age does psoriasis usually first make its appearance?

Most commonly between the ages of fifteen and thirty. It is rarely seen before the tenth year, and a first attack is uncommon after the age of forty.

Has psoriasis any special parts of predilection?

The extensor surfaces of the limbs, especially the elbows and knees, are favorite localities, and even when the eruption is more or less general, these regions are usually most conspicuously involved.

The face often escapes, and the palms and soles, likewise the nails, are rarely involved. In exceptional instances, the eruption is limited almost exclusively to the scalp.

Are there any constitutional or subjective symptoms in psoriasis?

There is no systemic disturbance; but a variable amount of itching may be present, although, as a rule, it is not a troublesome symptom.

Describe the clinical appearances of a typical, well developed case.

Twenty or a hundred or more lesions, varying in size from a pin-head to a silver dollar, are usually present. They are sharply defined against the sound skin, are reddish, slightly elevated and infiltrated, and more or less abundantly covered with whitish, grayish or mother-of-pearl colored scales. The patches are usually scattered over the general surface, but are frequently more numerous on the extensor surfaces of the arms and legs, especially about the elbows and knees. Several closely-lying lesions may coalesce and a large, irregular patch be formed; some of the patches, also, may be more or less circinate, the central portion having, in a measure or completely, disappeared.

Give the development and history of a single lesion.

Every single patch of psoriasis begins as a pin-point or pin-head-sized, hyperæmic, scaly, slightly-elevated lesion; it increases gradually, and in the course of several days or weeks usually reaches the size of a dime or larger, and then may remain stationary; or involution begins to take place, usually by a disappearance, partially or completely, of the central portion, and finally of the whole patch. [Pg 88]

Describe the so-called clinical varieties of psoriasis.

As clinically met with, the patches present are, as a rule, in all stages of development. In some instances, however, the lesions, or the most of them, progress no further than pin-head in size, and then remain stationary, constituting *psoriasis punctata*; in other cases, they may stop short after having reached the size of drops— *psoriasis guttata*; in others (and this is the usual clinical type) the patches develop to the size of coins—*psoriasis nummularis*. In some cases there is a strong tendency for the central part of the lesions to disappear, and the process then remain stationary, the patches being ring-shaped—*psoriasis circinata;* and occasionally several such rings coalesce, the coalescing portions disappearing and the eruption be more or less serpentine—*psoriasis gyrata*. Or, in other instances, several large contiguous lesions may coalesce and a diffused, infiltrated patch covering considerable surface results— *psoriasis diffusa, psoriasis inveterata*.

Fig. 17.

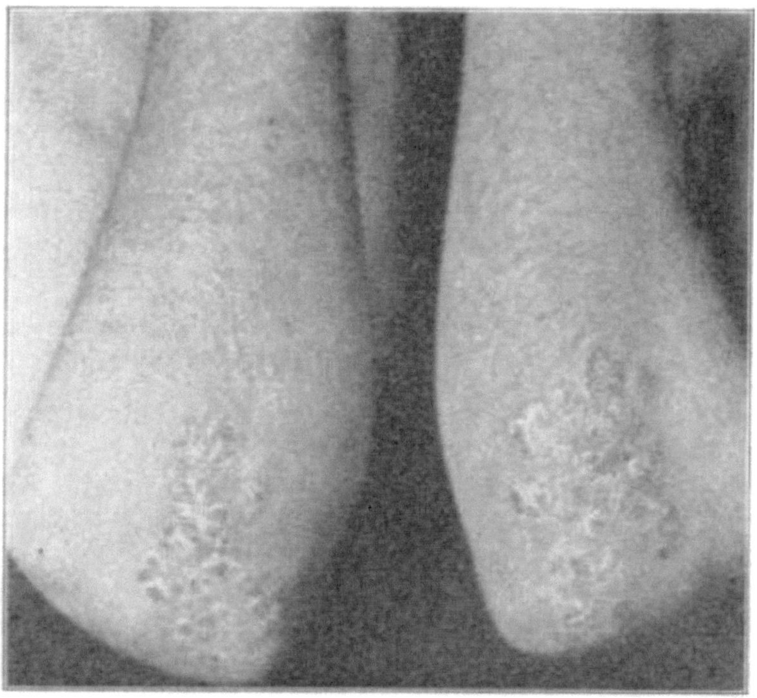

Psoriasis.

[Pg 89]

Is the eruption of psoriasis always dry?

Yes.

What course does psoriasis pursue?

As a rule, eminently chronic. Patches may remain almost indefinitely, or may gradually disappear and new lesions appear elsewhere, and so the disease may continue for months and, sometimes, for years; or, after continuing for a longer or shorter period, may subside and the skin remain free for several months or one or two years, and, in rare instances, may never return.

Fig. 18.

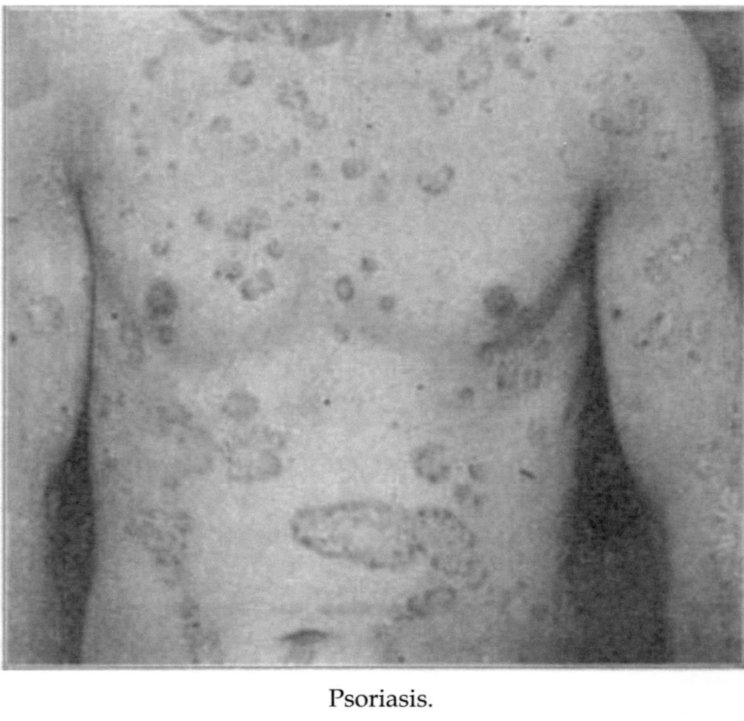

Psoriasis.

Is the course of psoriasis influenced by the seasons?

As a rule, yes; there is a natural tendency for the disease to become less active or to disappear altogether during the warm months. [Pg 90]

What is known in regard to the etiology of psoriasis?

The causes of the disease are always more or less obscure. There is often a hereditary tendency, and the gouty and rheumatic diathesis must occasionally be considered potential. In some instances it is apparently influenced by the state of the general health. It is a rather common disease and is met with in all walks of life.

Is psoriasis contagious?

No. In recent years the fact of its exhibiting a family tendency has been thought as much suggestive of contagiousness as of heredity.

What is the pathology?

According to modern investigations, it is an inflammation induced by hyperplasia of the rete mucosum; and it is beginning to be believed that this hyperplasia may have a parasitic factor as the starting-cause.

With what diseases are you likely to confound psoriasis?

Chiefly with squamous eczema and the papulo-squamous syphiloderm; and on the scalp, also with seborrhœa. It can scarcely be confounded with ringworm.

How is psoriasis to be distinguished from squamous eczema?

By the sharply-defined, circumscribed, scattered, scaly patches, and by the history and course of the individual lesions.

In what respects does the papulo-squamous syphiloderm differ from psoriasis?

The scales of the squamous syphilide are usually dirty gray in color and more or less scanty; the patches are coppery in hue, and usually several or more characteristic scaleless, infiltrated papules are to be found. The face, palms, and soles are often the seat of the syphilitic eruption; and, moreover, *concomitant symptoms of syphilis,* such as sore throat, mucous patches, glandular enlargement, rheumatic pains, falling out of the hair, together with the history of the initial lesion, are one, several, or all usually present.

How does seborrhœa differ from psoriasis?

Seborrhœa of the scalp is usually diffused, with but little redness and no infiltration; moreover, the scales of seborrhœa are greasy, dirty gray or brownish, while those of psoriasis are dry and [Pg 91] commonly whitish or mother-of-pearl colored. Psoriasis of the scalp rarely exists independently of other patches elsewhere on the general surface.

That variety of seborrhœa, commonly known as eczema seborrhoicum, presents at times, both on scalp and general surface, a strong resemblance to psoriasis, but the character of the scales and distribution of psoriasis, as above stated, are distinguishing points; seborrhœa, moreover, favors hairy surfaces and in extensive examples the scalp, eyebrows, sternal, and pubic regions rarely escape.

How does psoriasis differ from ringworm?

By its greater scaliness, by its higher degree of inflammatory action, and by its larger number of patches, as also by its history. In ringworm *all* the patches tend to clear up in the centre; in psoriasis this is rarely, if ever, so. If there is still any doubt, microscopic examination of the scrapings will determine.

Give the prognosis of psoriasis.

The prognosis is usually favorable, so far as concerns the immediate eruption, but as to recurrences, nothing positive can be stated. In rare instances, however, the cure remains permanent.

How is psoriasis treated?

Both constitutional and local remedies are demanded in most cases.

Do dietary measures exert any influence?

As a rule, no; but the food should be plain, and an excess of meat avoided.

Name the important constitutional remedies usually employed in psoriasis.

Arsenic is of first importance. It is not suitable in acute or markedly inflammatory types; but is most useful in the sluggish, chronic forms of the disease. The dose should never be pushed beyond slight physiological action. It may be given as arsenious acid in pill form, one-fiftieth to one-tenth of a grain three times daily, or as Fowler's solution, three to ten minims at a dose.

Alkalies, of which liquor potassæ is the most eligible. It is to be given in ten to twenty minim doses, largely diluted. It is valuable [Pg 92] in robust, plethoric, rheumatic or gouty individuals with psoriasis of an acute or markedly inflammatory type; it is not to be given to debilitated or anæmic subjects.

Salicin, sodium salicylate, and salophen in moderately full doses act well in some cases. Occasionally thyroid preparations have a good effect.

Potassium Iodide, in doses of thirty to one hundred grains, t.d., acts favorably in some instances; there are no special indications pointing toward its selection, unless it be the existence of a gouty or rheumatic diathesis.

Oil of copaiba, potassium acetate, oil of turpentine, oil of juniper, and other diuretics are valuable in some instances, and, while often failing, sometimes exert a rapid influence, especially in those cases in which the disease is extensive and inflammatory. Wine of antimony, given cautiously, is also sometimes of service in the acute inflammatory type in robust subjects.

Are such remedies as iron, quinine, nux vomica and cod-liver oil ever useful in psoriasis?

Yes. In debilitated subjects the administration of such remedies is at times attended with improvement in the cutaneous eruption.

What are the indications as regards the external measures?

Removal of the scales, and the use of soothing or stimulating applications, according to the individual case.

How are the scales removed?

In ordinary cases, either by warm, plain, or alkaline baths, or hot-water-and-soap washings; in those cases in which the scaling is abundant and adherent, washing with sapo viridis and hot water may be required. Baths of sal ammoniac, two to six ounces to the bath are also valuable in removing the scaliness. The tincture of green soap (tinctura saponis viridis) is especially valuable for cleansing purposes in psoriasis of the scalp. The hot vapor bath once or twice weekly is serviceable in keeping the scaliness in abeyance, and has, moreover, in some cases, a therapeutic value.

The frequency of the baths or washings will depend upon the rapidity with which the scales are reproduced. [Pg 93]

Are soothing applications often demanded in psoriasis?

In exceptional cases; in those in which the disease is acute, markedly inflammatory and rapidly progressing, mild, soothing applications must be temporarily employed, such as plain or bran baths, with the use of some bland oil or ointment. As a rule, however, the conditions, when coming under observation, are such as to permit of stimulating applications from the start. The most efficient soothing applications are the mild lotions and ointments employed in eczema of acute type.

How are the stimulating remedies employed in psoriasis applied?

As ointments, oils, and paints (pigmenta).

An ointment, if employed, is to be thoroughly rubbed in the diseased areas once or twice daily. The same may be said of the oily applications. The paints (medicated collodion and gutta-percha solution) are applied with a brush, once daily, or every second or third day, depending mainly upon the length of time the film remains intact and adherent.

Name the several important external remedies.

Chrysarobin, pyrogallol, tar, ammoniated mercury, β-naphthol, and resorcin.

Are these several external remedies equally serviceable in all cases?

No. Their action differs slightly or greatly according to the case and individual. A change from one to another is often necessary.

In what forms and strength are these remedies to be applied?

Chrysarobin is applied in several ways: as an ointment, twenty to sixty grains to the ounce, rubbed in once or twice daily; this is the most rapid but least cleanly and eligible method. As a pigment, or paint, as in the following:—

℞ Chrysarobini, ... ʒj Acidi salicylici, ... gr. xx Etheris, ... fʒj Ol. ricini, ... ℳx Collodii, ... fʒvij. M.

[Pg 94] Or it may be used in liquor gutta-perchæ (traumaticin), a drachm to the ounce. It may also be employed in chloroform, a drachm to the ounce; this is painted on, the chloroform evaporating, leaving a thin film of chrysarobin; over this is painted flexible collodion. If the patches are few and large, chrysarobin rubber-plaster may be used.

Chrysarobin is usually rapid in its effect, but it has certain disadvantages; it may cause an inflammation of the surrounding skin, and, if used near the eyes, may give rise to conjunctivitis. As a rule, it should not be employed about the head. Moreover, it stains the linen permanently and the skin temporarily.

Pyrogallol is valuable, and is employed in the same manner and strength as chrysarobin. In collodion it should at first not be used of greater strength than three to four per cent., as in this form pyrogallol sometimes acts with unexpected energy. It is less rapid than chrysarobin, but it rarely inflames the surrounding integument. It stains the linen a light brown, however, and is not to be used over an extensive surface for fear of absorption and toxic effect. Oxidized pyrogallic acid, a somewhat milder drug in its effect, has been highly commended, and has the alleged advantage of being free from toxic action.

Tar is, all things considered, the most important external remedy. It is comparatively slow in its action, but is useful in almost all cases. As employed usually it is prescribed in ointment form, either as the official tar ointment, full strength or weakened with lard or petrolatum. It may also be used as pix liquida, with equal part of alcohol. Or the tar oils, oil of cade (ol. cadini), and oil of birch (ol. rusci) may be employed, either as oily applications or incorporated with ointment or with alcohol. Liquor carbonis detergens, in ointment, one to three drachms to the ounce of simple cerate and lanolin is a mild tarry application which is often useful. In stubborn patches an occasional thorough rubbing with a mixture of equal parts of liquor carbonis detergens and Vleminckx's solution, followed by a mild ointment, sometimes proves of value. In whatsoever form tar is employed it should be thoroughly rubbed in, once or twice daily, the excess wiped off, and the parts then dusted with starch or similar powder.

Ammoniated mercury is applied in ointment form, twenty to sixty grains to the ounce. Compared to other remedies it is clean and free from staining, although, as a rule, not so uniformly efficacious. [Pg 95] It is especially useful for application to the scalp and exposed parts. It should not be used over extensive surface for fear of absorption.

β-Naphthol and *resorcin* are applied as ointments, thirty to sixty grains to the ounce, and as they are (especially the former) practically free from staining, may be used for exposed surfaces.

Gallacetophenone and aristol also act well in some cases, applied in five- to ten-per-cent. strength, as ointments.

In obstinate patches the *x*-ray may be resorted to, employing it with caution and in the same manner as in other diseases.

Pityriasis Rosea.

(*Synonym:* Pityriasis Maculata et Circinata.)

What do you understand by pityriasis rosea?

Pityriasis rosea is a disease of a mildly inflammatory nature, characterized by discrete, and later frequently confluent, variously sized, slightly raised scaly macules of a pinkish to rosy-red, often salmon-tinged, color.

Upon what part of the body is the eruption usually found?

The trunk is the chief seat of the eruption, although not infrequently it is more or less general.

Describe the symptoms of pityriasis rosea.

The lesions, which appear rapidly or slowly, are but slightly elevated, somewhat scaly, usually rounded, except when several coalesce, when an irregularly outlined patch results. At first they are pale or bright pink or reddish, later a salmon tint (which is often characteristic) is noticed. The scaliness is bran-like or flaky, of a dirty gray color, and, as a rule, less marked in the central portion; it is never abundant. The skin is rarely thickened, the process being usually exceedingly superficial.

What course does pityriasis rosea pursue?

The eruption makes its appearance, as a rule, somewhat rapidly, usually attaining its full development in the course of one or two weeks, and then begins gradually to decline, the whole process occupying one or two months.

To what is pityriasis rosea to be attributed?

The cause is not known; it is variously considered as allied to seborrhœa (eczema seborrhoicum), as being of a vegetable-parasitic [Pg 96] origin, and as a mildly inflammatory affection somewhat similar to psoriasis. It is not a frequent disease.

How is pityriasis rosea distinguished from ringworm, psoriasis and the squamous syphiloderm?

From ringworm, by its rapid appearance, its distribution, the number of patches, and, if necessary, by microscopic examination of the scrapings.

Psoriasis is a more inflammatory disease, is seen usually more abundantly upon the limbs, the scales are profuse and silvery, and the underlying skin is red and has a glazed look; moreover, psoriasis, as a rule, appears slowly and runs a chronic course.

The squamous syphiloderm differs in its history, distribution, and above all, by the presence of concomitant symptoms of syphilis, such as glandular enlargement, sore throat, mucous patches, rheumatic pains, and falling out of the hair.

State the prognosis of pityriasis rosea.

It is favorable, the disease tending to spontaneous disappearance, usually in the course of several weeks or one or two months.

What treatment is to be advised in pityriasis rosea?

Laxatives and intestinal antiseptics, and ointments of salicylic acid (5-15 grains to the ounce), of sulphur (10-40 grains to the ounce); or a compound ointment containing both these ingredients can be prescribed. The ointment base can be equal parts of white vaselin and cold cream; in some instances Lassar's paste (starch powder, zinc oxid powder, each, ʒij; vaselin, ʒiv) seems more satisfactory.

Dermatitis Exfoliativa.

(*Synonyms:* General Exfoliative Dermatitis; Recurrent Exfoliative Dermatitis; Desquamative Scarlatiniform Erythema; Acute General Dermatitis; Recurrent Exfoliative Erythema; Pityriasis Rubra.)

Describe dermatitis exfoliativa.

Dermatitis exfoliativa is an inflammatory disease of an acute type, characterized by a more or less general erythematous inflammation, in exceptional instances vesicular or bullous, with epidermic desquamation or exfoliation accompanying or following its development. Constitutional disturbance, which may be of a serious character, is [Pg 97] sometimes present. It is a rare and obscure affection, running its course usually in several weeks or months, but exhibiting a decided tendency to relapse and recurrence. In many cases it is persistently chronic, with exacerbations and remissions. In some instances it develops from a long-continued and more or less generalized eczema or psoriasis, and in exceptional cases it is started by the careless use of mercurial ointment and of chrysarobin ointment.

Fig. 19.

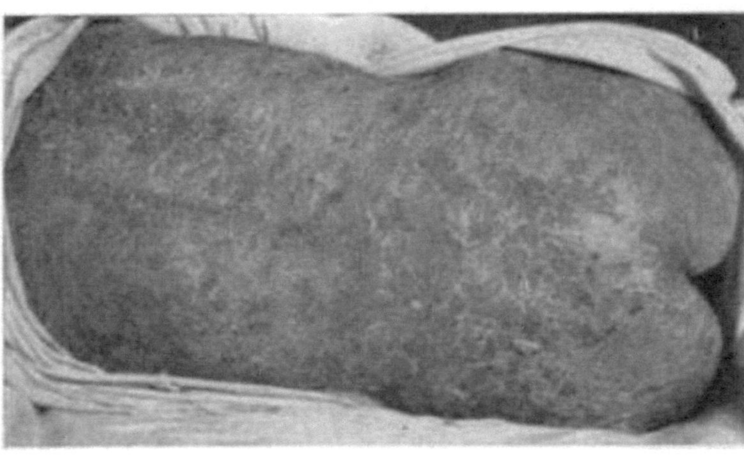

Dermatitis Exfoliativa.

In another type of the disease, formerly described as *pityriasis rubra*, the skin is pale red or violaceous-red, but is rarely thickened, continued exfoliation in the form of thin plates taking place. Its course is variable, lasting for years, with remissions.

An exfoliating generalized dermatitis is exceptionally observed in the first weeks of life (*dermatitis exfoliativa neonatorum*), lasting some weeks, and in most cases followed by recovery. There are no special constitutional symptoms, the fatal cases usually dying of marasmus.

As will be seen dermatitis exfoliativa varies considerably in degree; it may be extremely mild, resembling in appearance the scarlet-fever eruption (erythema scarlatiniforme) and running a rapid course; or the skin-condition and the systemic symptoms may be of grave and persistent character. [Pg 98]

Give the treatment of dermatitis exfoliativa.

General treatment is based upon indications, and externally soothing applications, such as are employed in acute and subacute eczema, are to be used.

Lichen Planus.

What is lichen planus?

Lichen planus is an inflammatory disease characterized by small, flat and angular, smooth and shining, or scaly, discrete or confluent, red or violaceous-red papules, having a distinctly papular or papulo-squamous course, and attended with more or less itching.

Describe the symptoms of lichen planus.

The eruption, as a rule, begins slowly, usually showing itself upon the extremities; the forearms, wrists and legs being favorite localities. It may appear as one or more groups or in the form of short or long bands. Occasionally its evolution is rapid and a considerable part of the surface may be invaded. The lesions are pin-head to small pea-sized, irregularly grouped or so closely crowded together as to form solid patches; they are quadrangular or polygonal in shape, usually flat, with central depression or umbilication, and are reddish or violaceous in color. At first they have a glazed or shining appearance; later, becoming slightly scaly, the scaliness being more marked where solid patches have resulted. New papules may appear from time to time, the older lesions disappearing and leaving persistent reddish or brownish pigmentation. Exceptionally the eruption presents in bands or lines, like rows of beads (*lichen moniliformis*). Very exceptionally a vesicular or bleb tendency in some of the lesions has been noted; doubtless, in most instances at least, this has been due to the arsenic so generally administered in this disease. In rare instances lichen planus lesions are also seen on the glans penis and on the buccal mucous membrane. In some cases, especially in the region of the ankle, the papules become quite large (*lichen planus hypertrophicus*), and in occasional cases there is a tendency in some of the lesions or patches to clear up centrally. There is, as a rule, considerable itching. There are no constitutional symptoms.

What is the etiology of lichen planus?

In some cases the disease is distinctly neurotic in character, in others no cause can be assigned. It is more especially met with at [Pg 99] middle age, and among the wealthier, professional, and luxurious classes.

Pathologically the first change noted in the epidermis is thought to be an acanthosis, followed by epithelial atrophy, and a hyperkeratosis, intercellular edema, and colloid degeneration of the prickle cells.

Does the disease bear any resemblance to the miliary papular syphilide, psoriasis, and papular eczema?

In some instances it does, but the irregular and angular outline, the slightly-umbilicated, flattened, smooth or scaly summits, and the dull-red or violaceous color, the history and course, of lichen planus, will serve to differentiate.

State the prognosis.

Under proper management the eruption, although often obstinate, yields to treatment.

What treatment would you prescribe in lichen planus?

A general tonic plan of medication is indicated in most cases, with such remedies as iron, quinine, nux vomica, and cod-liver oil and other nutrients. In many instances arsenic exerts a special influence, and should always be tried. Mercurials in moderate dosage have also a favorable action in most cases. Locally, antipruritic and stimulating applications, such as are used in the treatment of eczema, are to be employed, alkaline baths and tarry applications deserving special mention. Liquor carbonis detergens, applied weakened with several parts water, is a valuable application. In some cases, particularly if the disease is limited, external applications alone often suffice to bring about a cure.

Pityriasis Rubra Pilaris.

(*Synonyms:* Lichen Ruber; Lichen Ruber Acuminatus.)

Describe pityriasis rubra pilaris.

Pityriasis rubra pilaris is an extremely rare disease, usually of a mildly inflammatory nature, characterized by grayish, pale-red or reddish-brown follicular papules with somewhat hard or horny centres; discrete and confluent, and covering a part or the entire surface. The skin is harsh, dry and rough, feeling to the touch somewhat like the surface of a nutmeg-grater or a coarse file. More [Pg 100] or less scaliness is usually present in the confluent patches and on the palms and soles; in these latter regions the papules are rarely seen. The duration of the disease is variable, and relapses are common. It bears resemblance at times to keratosis pilaris, ichthyosis, dermatitis exfoliativa; it is considered identical with the lichen ruber acuminatus of Kaposi, and by many also with the lichen ruber of Hebra. The etiology is obscure.

Treatment, both constitutional and local, is to be based upon general principles; stimulating applications, with frequent baths, such as are advised in psoriasis, are the most satisfactory. It is rebellious, and not much more than palliation can be effected in some cases, in others the outlook is more hopeful.

Lichen Scrofulosus.

Describe lichen scrofulosus.

Lichen scrofulosus is a chronic, inflammatory disease, characterized by millet-seed-sized, rounded or flat, reddish or yellowish, more or less grouped, desquamating papules. The lesions have their start about the hair-follicles, occur usually upon the trunk, tend to group and form patches, and sooner or later become covered with minute scales. As a rule, there is no itching. It is a rare disease, and but seldom met with in America; it is seen chiefly in children and young people of a scrofulous diathesis. Scarring, slight in character, may or may not follow.

What is the treatment of lichen scrofulosus?

The condition responds to tonics and anti-strumous remedies.

Eczema.

(*Synonym:* Tetter; Salt Rheum.)

What is eczema?

An acute, subacute or chronic inflammatory disease, characterized in the beginning by the appearance of erythema, papules, vesicles or pustules, or a combination of these lesions, with a variable amount of infiltration and thickening, terminating either in discharge with the formation of crusts, in absorption, or in desquamation, and accompanied by more or less intense itching and a feeling of heat or burning. [Pg 101]

What are the several primary types of eczema?

Erythematous, papular, vesicular and pustular; all cases begin as one or more of these types, but not infrequently lose these characters and develop into the common clinical or secondary types—eczema rubrum and eczema squamosum.

Fig. 20.

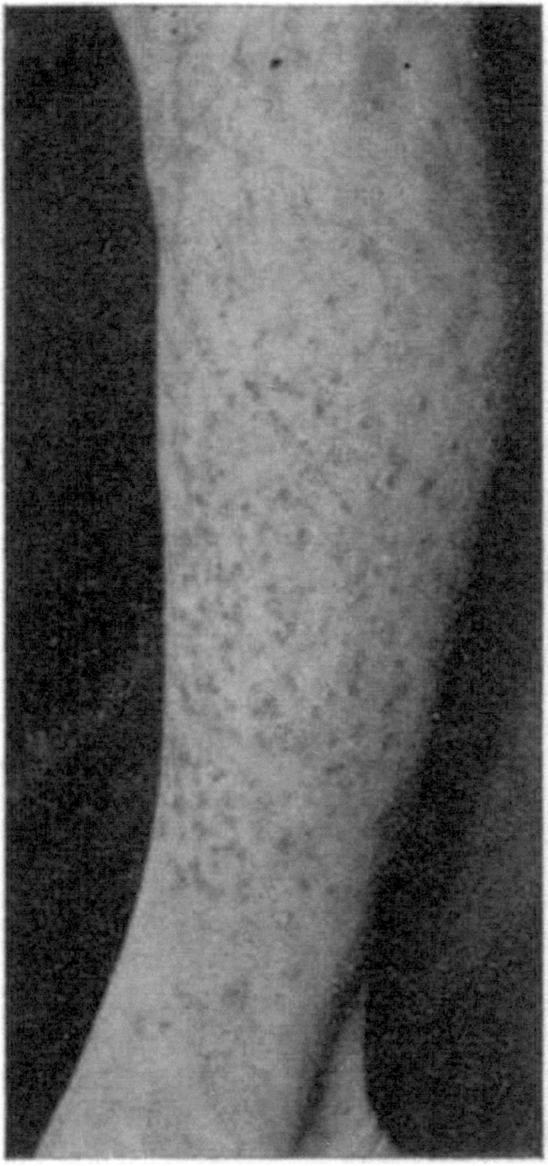

Papular Eczema (leg).

What other types are met with clinically?

Eczema rubrum, eczema squamosum, eczema fissum, eczema sclerosum and eczema verrucosum. Eczema seborrhoicum is probably a closely allied disease, occupying a middle position between ordinary eczema and seborrhœa. [Pg 102]

Describe the symptoms of erythematous eczema.

Erythematous eczema (*eczema erythematosum*) begins as one or more small or large, irregularly outlined hyperæmic macules or patches, with or without slight or marked swelling, and with more or less itching or burning. At first it may be ill-defined, but it tends to spread and its features to become more pronounced. It may be limited to a certain region, or it may be more or less general. When fully developed, the skin is harsh and dry, of a mottled, reddish or violaceous color, thickened, infiltrated and usually slightly scaly, with, at times, a tendency toward the formation of oozing areas. Punctate and linear scratch-marks may usually be seen scattered over the affected region.

Its most common site is the face, but it is not infrequent upon other parts.

Fig. 21.

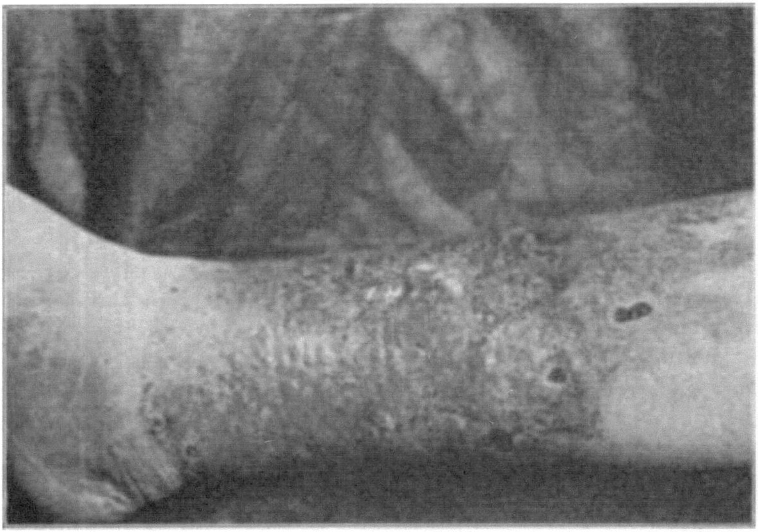

Eczema Rubrum.

What course does erythematous eczema pursue?

It tends to chronicity, continuing as the erythematous form, or the skin may become considerably thickened and markedly scaly, [Pg 103] constituting eczema squamosum; or a moist oozing surface, with more or less crusting, may take its place—eczema rubrum.

Describe the symptoms of papular eczema.

Papular eczema (*eczema papulosum*) is characterized by the appearance, usually in numbers, of discrete, aggregated or closely-crowded, reddish, pin-head-sized acuminated or rounded papules. Vesicles and vesico-papules are often intermingled. The itching is commonly intense, as often attested by the presence of scratch-marks and blood crusts.

It is seen most frequently upon the extremities, especially the flexor surfaces.

Fig. 22.

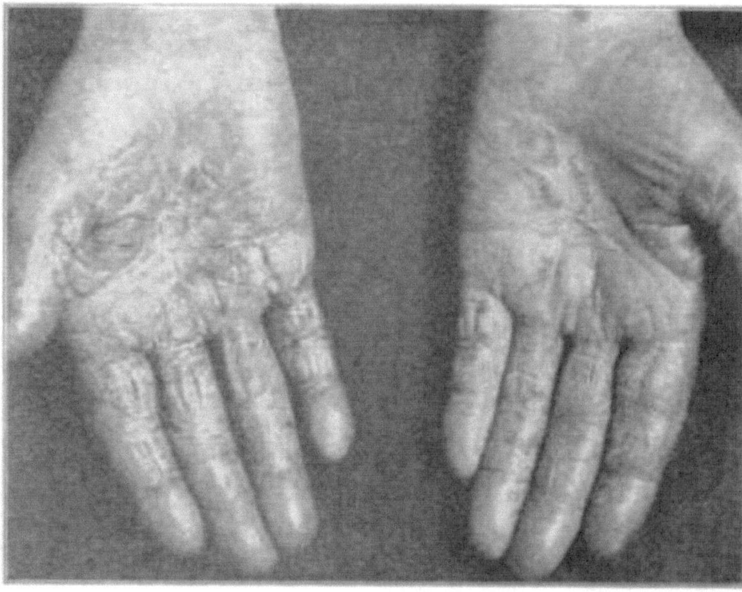

Eczema Squamosum et tissum.

What course does papular eczema pursue?

The lesions tend, sooner or later, to disappear, but are usually replaced by others, the disease thus persisting for weeks or months; in places where closely crowded, a solid, thickened, scaly sheet of eruption may result—eczema squamosum. [Pg 104]

Describe the symptoms of vesicular eczema.

Vesicular eczema (*Eczema vesiculosum*) usually appears, on one or several regions, as more or less diffused inflammatory reddened patches, upon which rapidly develop numerous closely-crowded pin-point to pin-head-sized vesicles, which tend to become confluent and form a solid sheet of eruption. The vesicles soon mature and rupture, the discharge drying to yellowish, honeycomb-like crusts. The oozing is usually more or less continuous, or the disease may decline, the crusts be cast off, to be quickly followed by a new crop of vesicles. In those cases in which the process is markedly acute, considerable swelling and œdema are present. Scattered papules, vesico-papules and pustules may usually be seen upon the involved area or about the border.

The face in infants (*crusta lactea*, or *milk crust*, of older writers), the neck, flexor surfaces and the fingers are its favorite localities.

What course does vesicular eczema pursue?

Usually chronic, with acute exacerbations. Not infrequently it passes into eczema rubrum.

Describe the symptoms of pustular eczema.

Pustular eczema (*eczema pustulosum, eczema impetiginosum*) is probably the least common of all the varieties. It is similar, although usually less actively inflammatory, in its symptoms to eczema vesiculosum, the lesions being pustular from the start or developing from preëxisting vesicles; not infrequently the eruption is mixed, the pustules predominating. There is a marked tendency to rupturing of the lesions, the discharge drying to thick, yellowish, brownish or greenish crusts.

Its most common sites are the scalp and face, especially in young people and in those who are ill-nourished and strumous.

What course does pustular eczema pursue?

Usually chronic, continuing as the same type, or passing into eczema rubrum.

Describe the symptoms of squamous eczema.

Squamous eczema (*eczema squamosum*) may be defined as a clinical variety, the chief symptoms of which are a variable degree of scaliness, more or less thickening, infiltration, and redness, with [Pg 105] commonly a tendency to cracking or fissuring of the skin, especially when the disease is seated about the joints. It is developed, as a rule, from the erythematous or papular type. Itching is slight or intense.

The disease is not uncommon upon the scalp.

What is the course of squamous eczema?

Essentially chronic.

Fig. 23.

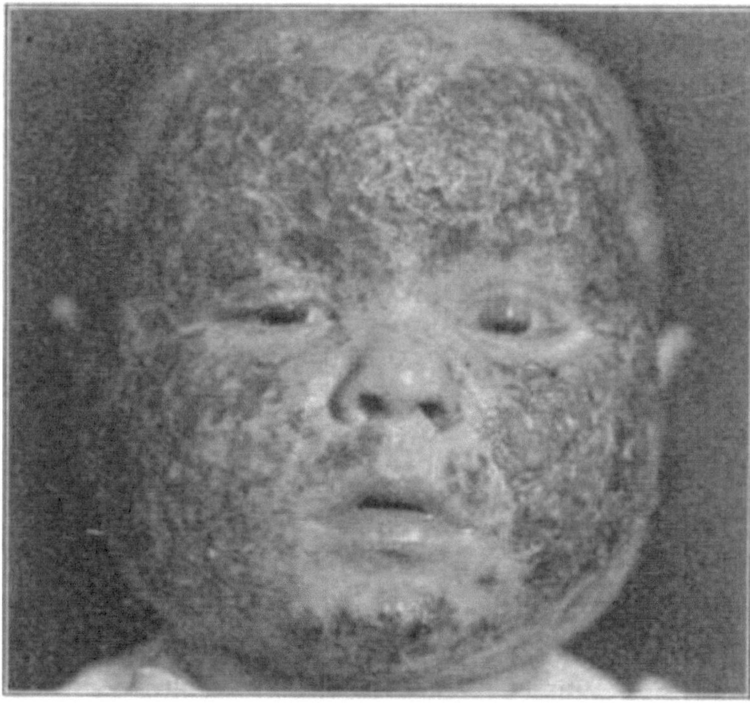

Eczema of the Face and Scalp.

Describe the symptoms of eczema rubrum.

Eczema rubrum is characterized by a red, raw-looking, weeping, oozing or discharging surface, attended with more or less inflammatory thickening, infiltration and swelling; the exudation, consisting of serum, sometimes bloody, dries into thick yellowish or reddish-brown crusts. At one time the whole diseased area may be hidden under a mass of crusting, at other times a red, raw-looking, weeping surface (*eczema madidans*) is the most striking feature. Itching is slight or intense, or the subjective symptom may be a feeling of [Pg 106] burning, It is an important clinical type, usually developing from the vesicular, pustular or other primary variety.

It is common about the face and scalp in children, and the middle and lower part of the leg in elderly people.

What is the course of eczema rubrum?

Chronic, varying in intensity from time to time.

Describe the symptoms of fissured eczema.

The conspicuous symptom is a marked tendency to fissuring or cracking of the skin (*eczema fissum; eczema rimosum*). This tendency is usually a part of an erythematous or squamous eczema, the fissuring constituting the most conspicuous and troublesome symptom. *Chapping* is an extremely mild but familiar example of this type.

It is especially common about the hands and fingers.

What is the course of fissured eczema?

It is more or less persistent, the tendency to fissuring varying considerably according to the state of the weather, often disappearing spontaneously in the summer months.

Describe eczema sclerosum and eczema verrucosum.

In eczema sclerosum the skin is thickened, infiltrated, hard, and almost horny. Eczema verrucosum presents similar conditions, but, in addition, displays a tendency to papillary or wart-like hypertrophy. In both varieties the disease is usually seated about the ankle or the foot, developing from the papular or squamous type. They are uncommon, and obstinately chronic.

State the nature of the subjective symptoms in eczema.

Itching, commonly intense, is usually a conspicuous symptom; it may be more or less paroxysmal. In some cases burning and heat constitute the main subjective phenomena.

Is eczema accompanied by febrile or systemic symptoms?

No. In rare instances, in acute universal eczema, slight febrile action, or other systemic disturbance, may be noted at the time of the outbreak. [Pg 107]

Is the eczematous eruption (patch or patches) sharply defined against the neighboring sound skin?

No. In almost all instances the diseased area merges gradually and imperceptibly into the surrounding healthy integument.

What is the character of eczema as regards the degree of inflammatory action?

The inflammatory action may be acute, subacute or sluggish in character, and may be so from the start and so continue throughout its whole course; or it may, as is usually the case, vary in intensity from time to time.

State the character of eczema as regards duration.

As a rule, it is a persistent disease, showing little, if any, tendency to spontaneous disappearance.

Is eczema influenced by the seasons?

Yes. With comparatively few exceptions the disease is most common and much worse in cold, windy, winter weather.

To what may eczema be ascribed?

Eczema may be due to constitutional or local causes, or to both. It may be considered, in fact, as a reaction of the skin tissues against some irritant, and the latter may have its origin from within or without.

Name some of the important constitutional or predisposing causes.

Gouty diathesis, rheumatic diathesis, disorders of the digestive tract, general debility or lack of tone, an exhausted state of the nervous system, dentition and struma.

Is a constitutional cause sufficient to provoke an attack?

Yes; but often the attack is brought about in those so predisposed by some local or external irritant.

Mention some of the external causes.

Heat and cold, sharp, biting winds, excessive use of water, strong soaps, vaccination, dyes and dyestuffs, chemical irritants, and the like. There is a growing belief that some cases presenting eczematous aspects are probably parasitic in origin. In fact, some observers hold to the microbic view of all cases of eczema. [Pg 108] Contact with the rhus plants, while producing a peculiar dermatitis, usually running an acute course terminating in recovery, may, in those predisposed, provoke a veritable and persistent eczema. In fact, in our examination as to causes in a given case, especially of the hands and face, all possible exciting factors should be inquired into, such as the handling of plants, chemicals, dyes, etc.

Fig. 24.

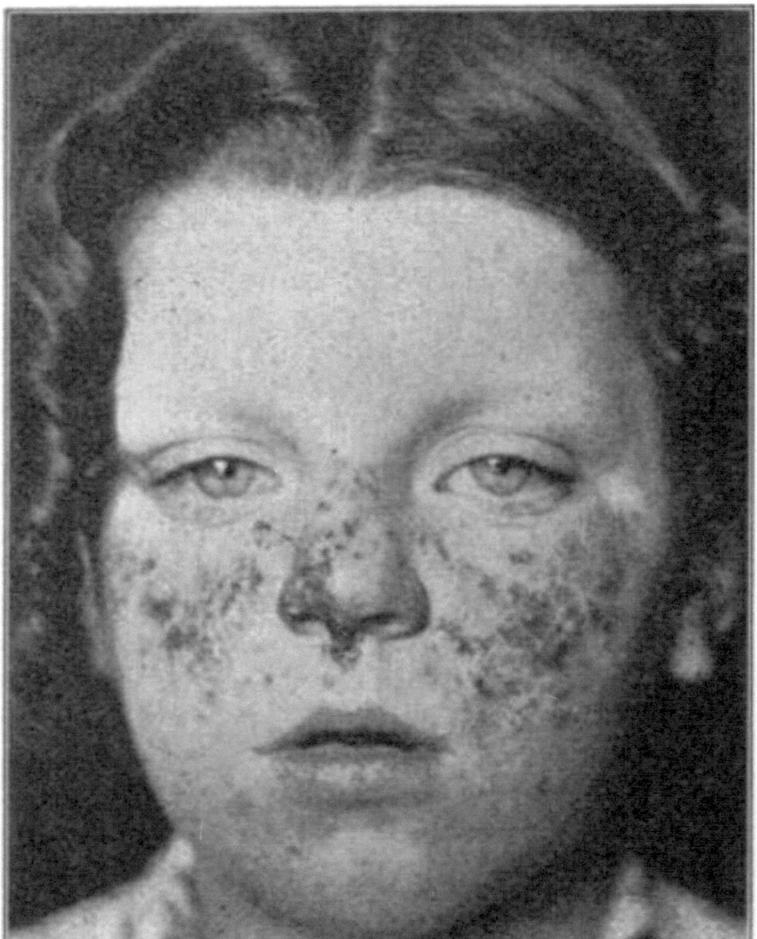

Eczema of Face.

Is eczema contagious?

No. The acceptance of a parasitic cause for the disease, however, necessarily carries with it the possibility of contagiousness under favoring conditions. Such is not supported, however, by practical experience. [Pg 109]

What is the pathology?

The process is an inflammatory one, characterized in all cases by hyperæmia and exudation, varying in degree according to the intensity and duration of the disease. The rete and papillary layer are especially involved, although in severe and chronic cases the lower part of the corium and even the subcutaneous tissue may share in the process.

Do the cutaneous manifestations of the eruptive fevers bear resemblance to the erythematous type of eczema?

Scarlatina and erysipelas may, to a slight extent, but the presence or absence of febrile and other constitutional symptoms will usually serve to differentiate.

What common skin diseases resemble some phases of eczema?

Psoriasis, seborrhœa, sycosis, scabies and ringworm.

How would you exclude psoriasis in a suspected case of eczema (squamous eczema)?

Psoriasis occurs in variously-sized, rounded, *sharply-defined* patches, usually scattered irregularly over the general surface, with special predilection for the elbows and knees. They are covered more or less abundantly with whitish, silvery or mother-of-pearl colored imbricated scales. The patches are always dry, and itching is, as a rule, slight, or may be entirely absent. Eczema, on the contrary, is often localized, appearing as one or more large, irregularly diffused patches; it merges imperceptibly into the sound skin, and there is often a history of characteristic serous or gummy oozing; the scaling is usually slight and itching almost invariably a prominent symptom.

How would you exclude seborrhœa (eczema seborrhoicum) in a suspected case of eczema?

Seborrhœa of the scalp is more commonly over the whole of that region and is relatively free from inflammatory symptoms; the scales are of a greasy character and the itching is usually slight or nil. On the other hand, in eczema of this region the parts are rarely invaded in their entirety; there may be at times the characteristic serous or gummy oozing; inflammatory symptoms are usually well-marked, the scales are dry and the itching is, as a rule, a prominent [Pg 110] symptom. These same differences serve to differentiate the diseases in other regions.

How does scabies differ from eczema?

Scabies differs from eczema in its peculiar distribution, the presence of the burrows, the absence of any tendency to patch formation, and usually by a clear history of contagion.

How would you exclude ringworm in a suspected case of eczema?

Ringworm is to be distinguished by its circular form, its fading in the centre, and in doubtful cases by microscopic examination of the scrapings.

How does eczema differ from sycosis?

Sycosis is limited to the hairy region of the face, is distinctly a follicular inflammation, and is rarely very itchy; eczema is diffused, usually involves other parts of the face, and itching is an annoying symptom.

State the general prognosis of eczema.

The disease is, under favorable circumstances, curable, some cases yielding more or less readily, others proving exceedingly rebellious. The length of time to bring about a result is always uncertain, and an opinion on this point should be guarded.

Upon what would you base your prognosis in the individual case?

The extent of disease, its duration and previous behavior, the removability of the exciting and predisposing causes, and the attention the patient can give to the treatment.

In eczema involving the lips, face, scrotum, and leg, and especially when this last-named exhibits a varicose condition of the veins, a cure is effected, as a rule, only through persistent and prolonged treatment.

Does eczema ever leave scars?

No. Upon the legs, in long-continued cases, more or less pigmentation usually remains.

How is eczema treated?

As a rule, eczema requires for its removal both constitutional and external treatment. [Pg 111] Certain cases, however, seem to be entirely local in their nature, and in these cases external treatment alone will have satisfactory results.

What general measures as to hygiene and diet are commonly advisable?

Fresh air, exercise, moderate indulgence in calisthenics, regular habits, a plain, nutritious diet; abstention from such articles of food as pork, salted meat, acid fruits, pastry, gravies, sauces, cheese, pickles, condiments, excessive coffee or tea drinking, etc. As a rule, also, beer, wine, and other stimulants are to be interdicted.

Upon what grounds is the line or plan of constitutional treatment to be based?

Upon indications in the individual case. A careful examination into the patient's general health will usually give the cue to the line of treatment to be adopted.

Mention the important remedies variously employed in the constitutional treatment.

Tonics—such as cod-liver oil, quinine, nux vomica, the vegetable bitters, iron, arsenic, malt, etc.

Alkalies—sodium salicylate, potassium bicarbonate, liquor potassæ, and lithium carbonate.

Alteratives—calomel, colchicum, arsenic, and potassium iodide.

Diuretics—potassium acetate, potassium citrate, and oil of copaiba.

Laxatives—the various salines, aperient spring waters, castor oil, cascara sagrada, aloes and other vegetable cathartics.

Digestives—pepsin, pancreatin, muriatic acid and the various bitter tonics.

Are there any remedies which have a specific influence?

No; although arsenic, in exceptional instances, seems to exert a special action. Cod-liver oil is also of great value in some cases.

Upon the whole the most important remedies are those which keep in view the maintenance of a proper and healthful condition of the gastro-intestinal tract, and especially with regular and rather free action of the bowels. [Pg 112]

In what class of cases does arsenic often prove of service?

In the sluggish, dry, erythematous, scaly and papular types.

In what cases is arsenic usually contraindicated?

It should never be employed in acute cases; nor in any instance (unless its action is watched), in which the degree of inflammatory action is marked, as an aggravation of the disease usually results.

What should be the character of the external treatment?

It depends mainly upon the degree of inflammatory action; but the stage of the disease, the extent involved, and the ability of the patient to carry out the details of treatment, also have a bearing upon the selection of the plan to be advised.

What is to be said about the use of soap and water in eczema?

In acute and subacute conditions soap and water are to be employed, as a rule, as infrequently and as sparingly as possible, as the disease is often aggravated by their too free use. Washing is necessary, however, for cleanliness and occasionally, also, for the removal of the crusts. On the other hand, in chronic, sluggish types the use of soap and water frequently has a therapeutic value.

How often should remedial applications be made?

Usually twice daily, although in some case, and especially those of an acute type, applications should be made every few hours.

Mention several remedies or plans of treatment to be used in the acute or actively inflammatory cases.

Black wash and oxide-of-zinc ointment conjointly, the wash thoroughly dabbed on, allowed to dry, the parts gently smeared with ointment; or the ointment may be applied spread on lint as a plaster.

Boric-acid wash (15 grains to the ounce) and oxide-of-zinc ointment, applied in the same manner as the above.

A lotion containing calamine and zinc oxide, the sediment drying and coating over the affected surface:—

> ℞ Calaminæ,
> Zinci oxidi, ...āā.................. ʒ ij-ʒ iij Glycerinæ, Alcoholis, ...āā................. fʒss Liq. calcis, ... f℥ij Aquæ, ... q.s. ... ad .... f℥vj. M.

[Pg 113] Another excellent lotion somewhat similar to the last, but of oily character, is made up of three drachms each of calamine and zinc oxide, one drachm of boric acid, ten to thirty drops of carbolic acid, and three ounces each of lime-water and oil of sweet almonds.

Carbolic-acid lotion, about two drachms to the pint of water, to which may be added two or three drachms each of glycerin and alcohol; or, if there is intense itching, carbolic acid may be added to the several washes already mentioned.

A lotion made of one or two drachms of liquor carbonis detergens [A] to four ounces of water.

The following wash, especially in the dry form of the disease:—

> ℞ Ac. borici, ... ʒiv Ac. carbolici, ... ʒj Glycerinæ, ... ʒij Alcoholis, ... ʒij Aquæ, ... q.s. ad. .... Oj. M.

[A] Liquor carbonis detergens is made by mixing together nine ounces of tincture soap bark and four ounces of coal tar, allowing to digest for eight days, and filtering. The tincture of soap bark used is made with one pound of soap bark to one gallon of 95 per cent. alcohol, digesting for a week or so. Instead of the proprietary name above, Prof. Duhring has suggested that of tinctura picis mineralis comp.

Dusting-powders, of starch, zinc oxide and Venetian talc, alone or severally combined, applied freely and often, so as to afford protection to the inflamed surface:—

℞ Talci venet, Zinci oxidi, ...āā.................... ʒiv Amyli, ... ℥j. M.

If washes or dusting-powders should disagree or are not desirable or practicable, ointments may be employed, such as—

Oxide-of-zinc ointment, cold cream, petrolatum, plain or carbolated, diachylon ointment (if fresh and well prepared), and a paste-like [Pg 114] ointment, as the following, usually called "salicylic-acid paste"; in markedly itchy cases, five to fifteen grains of carbolic may be added to each ounce:

℞ Ac. salicylici, ... gr. v-x Pulv. amyli, Pulv. zinci oxidi, ...āā.............. ʒij Petrolati, ... ʒiv M.

Or the following ointment:—

℞ Calaminæ, ... ʒj Ungt. zinci oxidi, ... ʒvij. M.

Name several external remedies and combinations useful in eczema of a subacute or mildly inflammatory type.

The various remedies and combinations useful when the symptoms are acute or markedly inflammatory (mentioned above), and more especially the several following:—

℞ Zinci oxidi, ... ʒij Liq. plumbi subacetat. dilut., ... fʒvj Glycerinæ, ... fʒij Infus. picis liq., ... f℥iij M.

A lotion containing resorcin, five to thirty grains to the ounce.

Solution of zinc sulphate, one-half to three grains to the ounce.

An ointment containing calomel or ammoniated mercury, as in the annexed formula:—

℞ Hydrargyri ammoniat. seu Hydrargyri chloridi mit., ... gr. x-xxx Ac. carbolici, ... gr. v-x Ungt. zinci oxidi, ... ℥j. M.

Another formula, more especially useful in eczema of the hands and legs, is the following:— [Pg 115]

℞ Ac. salicylici, ... gr. xxx Emp. plumbi, Emp. saponis, Petrolati, ...āā................. ℥j. M.

(This is to be applied as a plaster, spread on strips of lint, and changed every twelve or twenty-four hours.)

The paste-like ointment, referred to as useful in acute eczema, may also be used with a larger proportion (20 to 60 grains to the ounce) of salicylic acid.

The following, containing tar, may often be employed with advantage:—

℞ Ungt. picis liq., ... ʒj Ungt. zinci oxidi, ... ʒvij. M.

What is to be said in regard to the use of tarry applications?

Ointments or lotions containing tar should always be tried at first upon a limited surface, as occasionally skins are met with upon which this remedy acts as a more or less violent irritant. The coal tar lotion (liquor carbonis detergens) is the least likely to disagree and may be used as a mild ointment, one or two drachms to the ounce, or it may be diluted and used as a weak lotion as already referred to.

What external remedies are to be employed in eczema of a sluggish type?

The various remedies and combinations (mentioned above) useful in acute and subacute eczema may often be employed with benefit, but, as a rule, stronger applications are necessary, especially in the thick and leathery patches. The following are the most valuable:—

An ointment of calomel or ammoniated mercury; forty to sixty grains to the ounce.

Strong salicylic-acid ointment; a half to one drachm of salicylic acid to the ounce of lard.

Tar ointment, official strength; or the various tar oils, alone or with alcohol, as a lotion, or in ointment form. [Pg 116]

Liquor picis alkalinus [B] is a valuable remedy in chronic *thickened, hard* and *verrucous* patches, but is a strong preparation and must be used with caution. It is applied diluted, one part with from eight to thirty-two parts of water; or in ointment, one or two drachms to the ounce. In such cases, also, the following is useful:—

℞ Saponis viridis, Picis liq., Alcoholis, ...āā................. ʒiij. M. SIG. To be well rubbed in.

[B]

℞ Potassæ ,.. ʒj Picis liq., ... ʒij Aquæ, ... ʒv.

Dissolve the potash in the water, and gradually add to the tar in a mortar, with thorough stirring.

In similar cases, also, the parts may be thoroughly washed or scrubbed with sapo viridis and hot water until somewhat tender, rinsed off, dried, and a mild ointment applied as a plaster.

Lactic acid, applied with one to ten or more parts of water is also of value in the sclerous and verrucous types. Caustic potash solutions, used cautiously, may also be occasionally employed to advantage in these cases.

Another remedy of value in these cases, as well as in others of more or less limited nature, is the *x*-ray. Exposures every few days, of short duration and 4 to 10 inches distance, with medium vacuum tube. This method has served me well in occasional cases; caution is necessary, and it should not be pushed further than the production of the mildest reaction. The repeated application of a high-frequency current, by means of the vacuum electrodes, is a safer and sometimes an equally beneficial method.

Is there any method of treating eczema with fixed dressings?

Several plans have been advised from time to time; some are costly, and some require too great attention to details, and are therefore impracticable for general employment. The following are those in more common use:—

The *gelatin dressing*, as originally ordered, is made by melting over [Pg 117] a water-bath one part of gelatin in two parts of water—quickly painting it over the diseased area; it dries rapidly, and to prevent cracking glycerine is brushed over the surface. Or the glycerine may be incorporated with the gelatin and water in the following proportion: glycerine, one part; gelatin, four parts, and water eight parts. Medicinal substances may be incorporated with the gelatin mixture.

A good formula is the following:—

℞ Gelatin, ... ℥j Zinci oxidi,
.... ℥ss Glycerini, ... ℥iss
Aquæ, ... ℥ii-℥iij.

This should be prepared over a water-bath, and two per cent. ichthyol added. A thin gauze bandage can be applied to the parts over which this dressing is painted, before it is completely dry; it makes a comfortable fixed dressing and may remain on several days.

Plaster-mull and *gutta-percha plaster*. The plaster-mull, consisting of muslin incorporated with a layer of stiff ointment, and the gutta-percha plaster, consisting of muslin faced with a thin layer of India-rubber, the medication being spread upon the rubber coating.

Rubber plasters. These are medicated with the various drugs used in the external treatment of skin diseases, and are often of service in chronic patches.

Two new excipients for fixed dressings have recently been introduced—bassorin and plasment; the former is made from gum tragacanth, and the latter from Irish moss.

The following is a satisfactory formula for a tragacanth dressing:

> ℞ Tragacanth, ... gr. lxxv Glycerini, ... ♏ xxx Ac. carbolici, ... gr. x-xx Zinci oxidi, ... ʒiss-ʒiiss. M.

This is painted over the parts and allowed to dry, and a mild dusting powder sprinkled over. It cannot be used in warm weather or in folds, as it is apt to get sticky. The following is a bassorin paste which may be variously medicated. [Pg 118]

> ℞ Bassorin, ... ʒx Dextrin, ... ʒvj Glycerini, ... ℥ij. Aquæ, ... q.s. ad. ℥iij.

It should be prepared cold.

Another "drying dressing" which may be used in cool weather is:

> ℞ Zinci oxidi, ... ℥j Glycerini, ... ℥ss Mucilag. acaciæ, ... ℥ii-℥iv.

It may be variously medicated.

The plaster-mull is used in all types, especially the acute; the gelatin dressing, and the gutta-percha plaster, in the subacute and chronic; and the rubber plaster in chronic, sluggish patches only. Acacia, tragacanth, bassorin and plasment applications are used in cases of a subacute and chronic character.

Prurigo.

Define prurigo.

Prurigo is a chronic, inflammatory disease, characterized by discrete, pin-head- to small pea-sized, solid, firmly-seated, slightly raised, pale-red papules, accompanied by itching and more or less general thickening of the affected skin.

Describe the symptoms and course of prurigo.

The disease first appears upon the tibial regions, and its earliest manifestation may be urticarial, but there soon develop the characteristic small, millet-seed-sized, or larger, firm elevations, which may be of the natural color of the skin or of a pinkish tinge. The lesions, whilst discrete, are in great numbers, and closely crowded. The overlying skin is dry, rough and harsh; itching is intense, and, as a result of the scratching, excoriations and blood crusts are commonly present. In consequence of the irritation, the inguinal glands are enlarged. Sooner or later the integument becomes considerably thickened, hard and rough. Eczematous symptoms may be superadded. In severe cases the entire extensor surfaces of the legs and arms, and in some instances the trunk also, are invaded. It is worse in the winter season. [Pg 119]

What is known in regard to etiology and pathology?

It is a disease of the ill-fed and neglected, usually developing in early childhood, and persisting throughout life. It is extremely rare, even in its milder types, in this country. Clinically and pathologically it bears some resemblance to papular eczema.

Give the prognosis and treatment of prurigo.

The disease, in its severer types is, as a rule, incurable, but much can be done to alleviate the condition. Good, nourishing food, pure air and exercise are of importance. Tonics and cod-liver oil are usually beneficial. The local management is similar to that employed in chronic eczema. An ointment of β-naphthol, one-half to five per cent. strength, is highly extolled.

Acne.

Give a definition of acne.

Acne is an inflammatory, usually chronic, disease of the sebaceous glands, characterized by papules, tubercles, or pustules, or a mixture of these lesions, and seated usually about the face.

At what age does acne usually occur?

Between the ages of fifteen and thirty, at which time the glandular structures are naturally more or less active.

Describe the symptoms of acne.

Irregularly scattered over the face, and in some cases also over the neck, shoulders and upper part of the trunk, are to be seen several, fifty or more, pin-head- to pea-sized papules, tubercles or pustules; commonly the eruption is of a mixed type (*acne vulgaris*), the several kinds of lesions in all stages of evolution and subsidence presenting in the single case. Interspersed may generally be seen blackheads, or comedones. The lesions may be sluggish in character, or they may be markedly inflammatory, with hard and indurated bases. In the course of several days or weeks, the papules and tubercles tend gradually to disappear by absorption; or, and as commonly the case, they become pustular, discharge their contents, or dry and slowly or rapidly disappear, with or without leaving a permanent trace, new lesions arising, here and there, to take their place. In exceptional instances the eruption is limited to the back, and in these [Pg 120] cases the eruption is usually extensive and persistent, and not infrequently leaves scars.

What do you understand by acne punctata, acne papulosa, acne pustulosa, acne indurata, acne atrophica, acne hypertrophica, and acne cachecticorum?

These several terms indicate that the lesions present are, for the most part, of one particular character or variety.

Describe the lesions giving rise to the names of these various types.

Blocking up of the outlet of the sebaceous gland (comedo), which is usually the beginning of an acne lesion, may cause a moderate degree of hyperæmia and inflammation, and a slight elevation, with a central yellowish or blackish point results—the lesion of *acne punctata;* if the inflammation is of a higher grade or progresses, the elevation is reddened and more prominent—*acne papulosa;* if the inflammatory action continues, the interior or central portion of the papule suppurates and a pustule results—*acne pustulosa;* the pustule, in some cases, may have a markedly inflammatory and hard base—*acne indurata;* and not infrequently the lesions in disappearing may leave a pit-like atrophy or depression—*acne atrophica;* or, on the contrary, connective-tissue new growth may follow their disappearance—*acne hypertrophica;* and, in strumous or cachectic individuals, the lesions may be more or less furuncular in type, often of the nature of dermic abscesses, usually of a cold or sluggish character, and of more general distribution—*acne cachecticorum.*

What is acne artificialis?

Acne artificialis is a term applied to an acne or acne-like eruption produced by the ingestion of certain drugs, as the bromides and iodides, and by the external use of tar; this is also called *tar acne.*

What course does acne pursue?

Essentially chronic. The individual lesions usually run their course in several days or one or two weeks, but new lesions continue to appear from time to time, and the disease thus persists, with more or less variation, for months or years. In many cases there is, toward the age of twenty-five or thirty, a tendency to spontaneous disappearance of the disease.

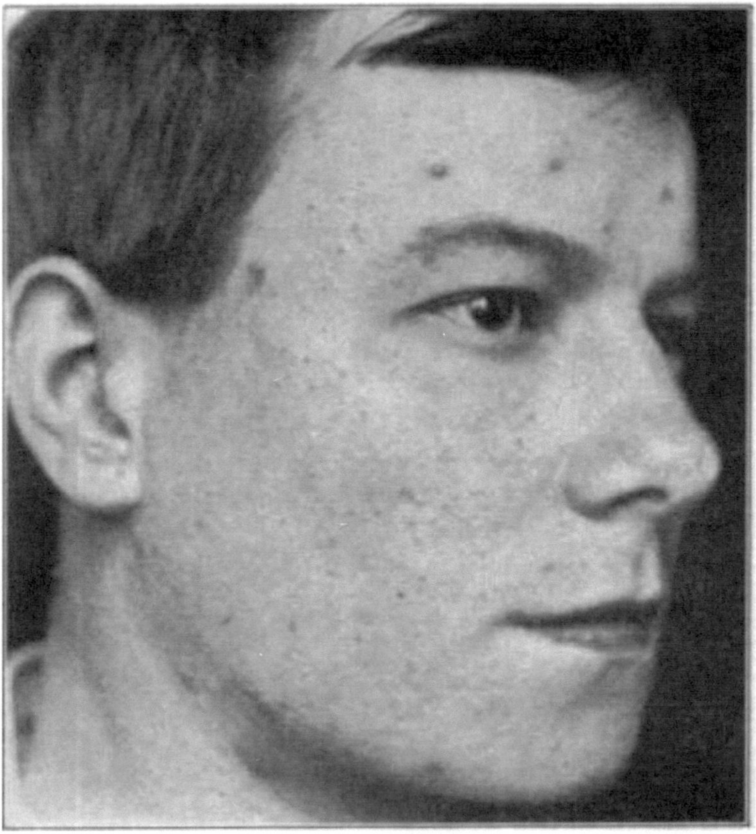

Acne

[Pg 121]

Is the eruption in acne usually abundant?

It varies in different cases and at different periods in the same case. In some instances, not more than five or ten papules and pustules are present at one time; in others they may be numerous. Not infrequently several lesions make their appearance, gradually run their course, and the face continues free for days or one or two weeks.

Does the eruption in acne disappear without leaving a trace?

In many instances no permanent trace remains, but in others slight or conspicuous scarring is left to mark the site of the lesions.

Are there any subjective symptoms in acne?

As a rule, not; but markedly inflammatory lesions are painful.

State the immediate or direct cause of an acne lesion.

Hypersecretion or retention of sebaceous matter. Recent investigations point to the possibility of a special bacillus being the exciting cause, in some instances at least. The pyogenic cocci are added factors in the pustular and furuncular cases.

Name the indirect or predisposing causes of acne.

Digestive disturbance, constipation, menstrual irregularities, chlorosis, general debility, lack of tone in the muscular fibres of the skin, scrofulosis; and medicinal substances such as the iodides and bromides internally, and tar externally.

Working in a dusty or dirty atmosphere is often influential, resulting in a blocking-up of the gland ducts. Workmen in paraffin oils or other petroleum products often present a furuncle-like acne.

The disease is more common in individuals of light complexion.

Is there any difficulty in the diagnosis of acne?

Not if it be remembered that acne eruption is limited to certain parts and is always follicular, and that the several stages, from the comedo to the matured lesion, are usually to be seen in the individual case.

In what respect does the pustular syphiloderm differ from acne?

By its general distribution, the longer duration of the individual lesions, the darker color, and the presence of concomitant symptoms of syphilis. [Pg 122]

What is the pathology of acne?

Primarily, acne is a folliculitis, due to retention or decomposition of the sebaceous secretion or to the introduction of a micro-organism; subsequently, the tissue immediately surrounding becoming involved, with the possible destruction of the sebaceous follicle as a result. The degree of inflammatory action determines the character of the lesions.

State the prognosis of acne.

It is usually an obstinate disease, but curable. Some cases yield readily, others are exceedingly rebellious, especially acne of the back. Success depends in a great measure upon a recognition and removal of the predisposing condition. Treatment is ordinarily a matter of months.

What measures of treatment are usually demanded in acne?

Constitutional and local measures; the former when indicated, the latter always.

Upon what is the constitutional treatment based?

Upon indications. Diet and hygienic measures are important.

In dyspepsia and constipation, bitter tonics, alkalies, acids, pepsin, saline and vegetable laxatives, are variously prescribed. Special mention may be made of the following:—

> ℞ Ext. rhamni pursh. fl., ... fʒij-fʒiv Tinct. nucis vom., ... fʒiij Tinct. cardamomi comp., ... q.s. ad. ℥iij. M. SIG.—fʒ t.d.

Or Hunyadi Janos or Friedrichshall water may be employed for a laxative purpose.

In chlorotic and anæmic cases the ferruginous preparations are of advantage. Cod-liver oil is often a remedy of great value, and is especially useful in strumous and debilitated subjects. Calx sulphurata in pill form, one-tenth to one-fourth grain four or five times daily, is said, acts well in the pustular variety. In some instances, more particularly in sluggish papular acne, arsenic, especially the sulphide of arsenic, acts favorably. Upon the whole, the line of

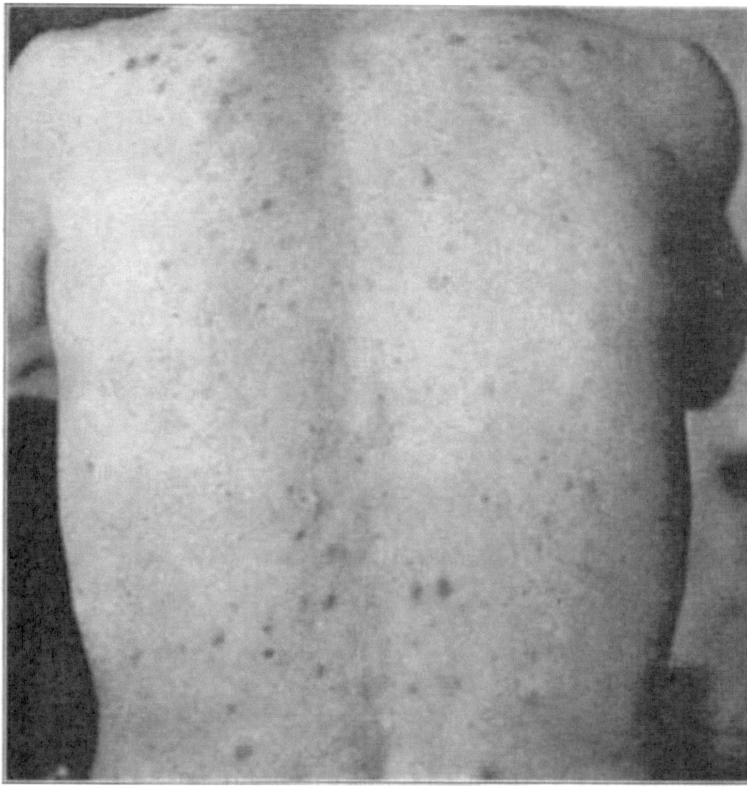

Acne of back [Pg 123]

treatment that keeps in view proper and healthy action of the gastro-intestinal canal is the most successful.

In inflammatory cases occurring in robust individuals the following is often of service:—

℞ Potassii acetat., ... ʒiv Liq. potassæ, ... fʒij Liq. ammonii acetat., ... q.s. ad. ..... f℥iij. M. SIG.—fʒj-fʒij t.d., largely diluted.

State the character of the local treatment in acne.

This must vary somewhat with the local conditions. Cases which are acute in character, in the sense that the lesions are markedly hyperæmic, tender and painful, require milder applications, and in exceptional instances soothing remedies are to be prescribed. As a rule, however, stimulating applications may be employed from the start.

The remedies are, for obvious reasons, most conveniently applied at bedtime.

What preliminary measures are to be advised in ordinary acne cases?

Washing the parts gently or vigorously, according to the irritability of the skin, with warm water and soap; subsequently rinsing, and sponging for several minutes with hot water, and rubbing dry with a soft towel; after which the remedial application is made. In sluggish and non-irritable cases sapo viridis or its tincture may often be advantageously used in place of the ordinary toilet soap.

The blackheads, so far as practicable, are to be removed by pressure with the fingers or with a suitable instrument (see Comedo), and the superficial pustules punctured and the contents pressed out. Scraping the affected parts with a blunt curette is a valuable measure, but is temporarily disfiguring. As a rule, however, cases do just as well without puncturing and scraping, and these methods sometimes leave behind scarring.

State the methods of external medication commonly employed.

By ointments and lotions. If an ointment is used, it is to be thoroughly rubbed in, in small quantity; if a lotion is employed, it [Pg 124] is to be well shaken, the parts freely dabbed with it for several minutes and then allowed to dry on.

State the object in view in local medication.

To hasten the maturation and disappearance of the existing lesions, and to stimulate the skin and glands to healthy action.

If slight irritation or scaliness results, the application is to be intermitted one or two nights; in the meantime nothing except the hot-water sponging, with or without the application of a mild soothing ointment, is to be employed.

Is it usually necessary to change from one external remedy to another in the course of treatment?

Yes. After a certain time one remedy, as a rule, loses its effect, and a change from lotion to ointment or the reverse, and from one lotion or ointment to another, will often be found necessary in order to bring about continuous improvement.

Name the various important remedies and combinations employed in the external treatment of acne.

Sulphur is the most valuable. It may often be applied with benefit as a simple ointment:—

℞ Sulphur, præcip., ... ʒss-ʒj Adipis benz. Lanolin, ...āā.................. ʒij.

Or it may be used as a lotion, as in the annexed formula:—

℞ Sulphur, præcip., ... ʒiss Pulv. tragacanthæ, ... gr. x1 Pulv. camphoræ, ... gr. xx Liq. calcis,........ q.s. ad. .... f℥iv. M.

Another lotion, especially useful in those cases in which an oily condition of the skin is present, is the following:—

℞ Sulphur, præcip., ... ʒiss Etheris, ... fʒiv Alcoholis, ... f℥iijss. M.

A compound lotion containing sulphur in one of its combinations is also valuable in many cases:— [Pg 125]

℞ Zinci sulphatis, Potassii sulphureti, ...āā........... ʒss-ʒiv Aquæ, ... ℥iv. M.

(The salts should be dissolved separately and then mixed; reaction takes place and the resulting lotion, when shaken, is milky in appearance, and free from odor; allowed to stand the particles settle, the sediment constituting about one-fourth to three-fourths of the whole bulk).

At times the addition to this formula of several drachms of alcohol and of five to ten minims of glycerin is of advantage.

An external remedy, often valuable, is ichthyol. It is thus prescribed:—

℞ Ichthyol, ... ʒss-ʒj Cerat. simp., ... ʒiv. M.

The various mercurial ointments, especially one of white precipitate, five to fifteen per cent. strength, are sometimes beneficial.

A compound lotion, containing mercury, which frequently proves serviceable, is:—

℞ Hydrarg. chlorid. corros., ... gr. ii-viij Zinci sulphatis, ... gr. x-xx Tinct. benzoini, ... fʒij Aquæ, ... q.s. ad. .... f℥iv.

In extremely sluggish cases the following, used cautiously, is of value:—

℞ Ichthyol, Saponis viridis, Sulphur, præcip., Lanolin, ...āā................ ʒj.

In such instances the application of a strong alcoholic resorcin lotion, ten to twenty-five per cent. strength, repeated several times daily till marked irritation and exfoliation occur (a matter usually of one to three days), will sometimes be followed by marked improvement. Acne of the back is treated with the same applications, but usually stronger; in this region applications of Vleminckx's [Pg 126] solution and formaldehyde solution, weakened considerably, at first at least, prove of value.

Obstinate and indurated lesions may be incised, the contents pressed out, and the interior touched with carbolic acid by means of a pointed stick. The *x*-ray has proved a most valuable addition to our resources in the treatment of acne, and is especially serviceable in extensive and obstinate cases. An exposure should be made about twice weekly, at a distance of five to ten inches and for from three to ten minutes, and a tube of medium vacuum used. It must be used with great caution and never beyond the production of the mildest erythema. The hair, eyes, and lips should be protected. The x-ray treatment is best reserved for obstinate cases, and then used mildly, and rather as an adjuvant to the ordinary methods than as the sole measure.

What precaution is to be taken in advising a change from a sulphur to a mercurial preparation or the reverse?

Several days should be allowed to intervene, otherwise a disagreeable, although temporary, staining or darkening of the skin results—from the formation of the black sulphuret of mercury.

Acne Rosacea.

Give a descriptive definition of acne rosacea.

Acne rosacea is a chronic, hyperæmic or inflammatory disease, limited to the face, especially to the nose and cheeks, characterized by redness, dilatation and enlargement of the bloodvessels, more or less acne and hypertrophy.

Describe the symptoms of acne rosacea.

The disease may be slight or well-marked. Redness, capillary dilatation, and acne lesions seated on the nose and cheeks, and sometimes on chin and forehead also, constitute in most cases the entire symptomatology.

A mild variety consists in simple redness or hyperæmia, involving the nose chiefly and often exclusively, and is to be looked upon as a passive congestion; this is not uncommon in young adults and is often associated with an oily seborrhœa of the same parts. In many [Pg 127] cases the condition does not progress beyond this stage. In other cases, however, sooner or later the dilated capillaries become permanently enlarged (*telangiectasis*) and acne lesions are often present— constituting the middle stage or grade of the disease; this is the type most frequently met with. In exceptional instances, still further hypertrophy of the bloodvessels ensues, the glands are enlarged, and a variable degree of connective-tissue new growth is added; this latter is usually slight, but may be excessive, the nose presenting an enlarged and lobulated appearance (*rhinophyma*).

Fig. 25.

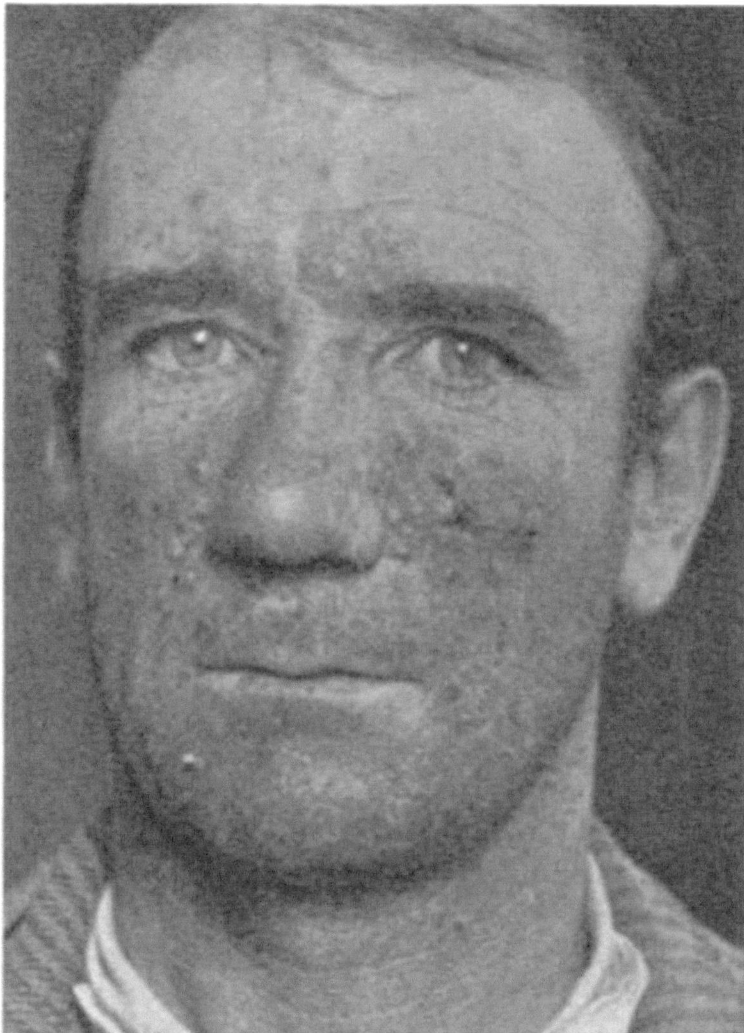

Acne Rosacea.

[Pg 128]

Are there any subjective symptoms in acne rosacea?

As a rule, no. Some of the acne lesions may be tender and painful, and at times there is a feeling of heat and burning.

What do you know in regard to the etiology?

In many cases the causes are obscure. Chronic digestive and intestinal disorders, anæmia, chlorosis, continued exposure to heat or cold, menstrual and uterine irregularities, and the too free use of spirituous liquors, tea, etc. are often responsible factors.

It is essentially a disease of adult life, common about middle age, occurring in both sexes, but rarely reaching the same degree of development in women as observed at times in men.

Is acne rosacea easily recognized?

Yes. The redness, acne lesions, dilated capillaries, and, at times, the glandular and connective-tissue hypertrophy; the limitation of the eruption to the face, especially the region of the nose; the evident involvement of the sebaceous glands, the absence of ulceration, taken with the history of the case, are characteristic.

It is to be distinguished from the tubercular syphiloderm and lupus vulgaris, diseases to which it may bear rough resemblance.

State the prognosis of acne rosacea.

All cases may be favorably influenced by treatment; the mild and moderately-developed types are, as a rule, curable, but usually obstinate. It is a persistent disease, showing little, if any, tendency to disappear spontaneously.

What is the method of treatment?

Both constitutional and local measures are demanded in most cases.

Upon what is the constitutional treatment to be based?

The constitutional treatment, beyond a regulation of the diet, is to be based upon a correct appreciation of the etiological factors in the individual case. There are no special remedies. Iron, cod-liver oil, tonics, ergot, alkalies, saline laxatives, and similar drugs are to be variously prescribed.

What is the external treatment?

In many respects, both as to the preliminary measures and remedies, [Pg 129] essentially the same as that employed in the treatment of simple acne (*q. v.*). The *x*-ray treatment is not so efficient in this disease, however, as in acne. In addition to the treatment there found, several other applications deserve mention:—

In many cases *Vleminckx's solution* [C] is valuable, applied diluted with one to ten parts of water. Also, a mucilaginous paste containing sulphur:—

> ℞ Mucilag. acaciæ, ... fʒiij Glycerinæ, ... fʒij Sulphur, præcip., ... ʒiij. M.

[C]

> ℞ Calcis, ... ℥ss Sulph. sublimat., ... ℥j Aquæ, ... ℥x.

To be boiled down to ℥vj and filtered.

Or a similar paste with the glycerine in the foregoing replaced with ichthyol may be used.

In what manner are the dilated bloodvessels and connective-tissue hypertrophy to be treated?

The enlarged capillaries are to be destroyed by incision or by electrolysis. Properly managed the vessels may be thus destroyed, but unless the predisposing causes have disappeared or have been remedied, a new growth may take place.

If the knife is employed, the vessels are either slit in their length or cut transversely at several points. The method by electrolysis is the same as used in the removal of superfluous hair (*q. v.*).; the needle may, if the vessel is short, be inserted along its calibre, or if long, may be inserted at several points in its length.

Excessive connective-tissue growth, exceptionally met with, is to be treated by ablation with the scissors or knife.

Acne Varioliformis.

(*Synonyms:* Acne Frontalis; Acne Rodens; Acne Necrotica; Lupoid Acne; Necrotic Granuloma.)

Describe acne varioliformis.

Acne varioliformis is characterized by lesions of a moderately superficial papulo-pustular type, which in disappearing leave slight or [Pg 130] well-marked pit-like scars. The forehead and scalp are the favorite sites, but they may also occur elsewhere. The eruption is rather scanty as a rule, consisting usually of ten to thirty lesions. They begin as small maculo-papules, as papules, or as minute nodules in or on the skin, and gradually become small pea-sized, with a tendency to slight vesiculation or pustulation at the central part. The lesion is sluggish in its course, drying to a thin crust, which finally falls off, leaving a depressed variola-like scar. New lesions arise from time to time, and the disease thus continues almost indefinitely. There may or may not be itching. In what appears to be a variety of this disease, known usually as *acne urticata,* there is considerable itching just at the time the lesion is appearing. The malady is not frequent, but occurs in both sexes, usually in those between the ages of twenty and fifty. It seems probable that the eruption is parasitic in origin.

The maladies variously known as hydradenitis suppurativa, acnitis, spiradenitis, folliclis, granuloma necroticum, etc., in which the lesions, primarily at least, are somewhat deeper seated, sluggish in their course, and followed by scarring, could be also included under this head.

Give the prognosis and treatment.

The disease is rebellious and tends to recur. The most efficient applications are those of sulphur and resorcin, the same as prescribed in ordinary acne.

Sycosis.

(*Synonyms:* Sycosis Vulgaris; Sycosis Non-parasitica; Folliculitis Barbæ; Sycosis Coccogenica.)

What do you understand by sycosis?

Sycosis is a chronic, inflammatory affection involving the hair-follicles, usually of the moustache and bearded regions only, and characterized by papules, tubercles, and pustules perforated by hairs.

Describe the symptoms of sycosis.

Sycosis begins by the formation of papules and pustules about the hair-follicles; the lesions occur in numbers, in close proximity, [Pg 131] and together with the accompanying inflammation, make up a small or large area. The pustules are small, rounded, flat or acuminated, discrete, and yellowish in color; they are perforated by hairs, show no tendency to rupture, and are apt to occur in crops, drying to thin yellowish or brownish crusts. Papules and tubercles are often intermingled. More or less swelling and infiltration are noticeable.

Fig. 26.

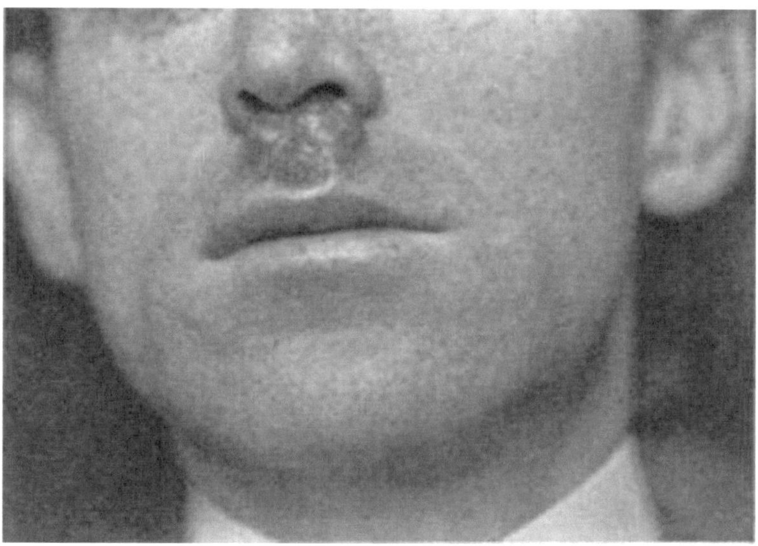

Sycosis—not infrequently begins in, and sometimes limited to, this region.

The disease is seen, as a rule, only on the bearded part of the face, either about the cheeks, chin or upper lip, involving a small portion or the whole of these parts. It is also sometimes met with involving the hair follicles just within the nasal orifice, and may even be limited to this region.

Occasionally a sycosiform eruption, usually of the side of the bearded region, leaves behind a smooth or keloidal scar, the disease gradually extending—*ulerythema sycosiforme* (lupoid sycosis).

An inflammation of the hair-follicles of the scalp apparently sycosiform in character, occurring as discrete or aggregated lesions, is sometimes observed, the follicles being destroyed and atrophy or slight scarring resulting—*folliculitis decalvans*.

Does conspicuous hair loss occur in sycosis?

Ordinarily not; the hairs are, especially at first, usually firmly seated, but in those cases in which suppuration is active, and has [Pg 132] involved the follicles, they may, as a rule, be easily extracted. In some cases destruction of the follicles ensues and slight scarring and permanent hair loss result.

State the character of the subjective symptoms.

Pain and itching and a sense of burning, variable as to degree, may be present.

What is the course of the disease?

Essentially chronic, the inflammatory action being of a subacute or sluggish character, with acute exacerbations.

State the causes of sycosis.

Upon the upper lip it may have its origin in a nasal catarrh. Entrance into the follicles of pyogenic micrococci is now regarded as the essential factor. This view being accepted, carries with it the possibility of contagiousness.

It is seen in the male sex only, usually in those between the ages of twenty-five and fifty; and is met with in those in good and bad health, and among rich and poor. It is comparatively infrequent.

What is the pathology of sycosis?

The disease is primarily a perifolliculitis, the follicle and its sheath subsequently becoming involved in the inflammatory process.

How would you distinguish sycosis from eczema?

Eczema is rarely sharply limited to the bearded region, but is apt to involve other parts of the face; moreover, the lesions are usually confluent, and there is either an oozing, red crusted surface, or it is dry and scaly.

How would you exclude tinea sycosis in the diagnosis?

In tinea sycosis, or ringworm sycosis, the history of the case is different. The parts are distinctly lumpy and nodular; the hairs are soon involved and become dry, brittle, loose, and fall out, or they may be readily extracted. The superficial type of ringworm sycosis is readily distinguished by the ring-like character of the patches. In doubtful cases, microscopic examination of the hairs may be resorted to.

Give the prognosis of sycosis.

The disease is curable, but almost invariably obstinate and rebellious to treatment. The duration, extent, and character of the [Pg 133] inflammatory process must all be considered. An expression of an opinion as to the length of time required for a cure should always be guarded.

Ulerythema sycosiforme is extremely obstinate. Folliculitis decalvans is also rebellious.

How is sycosis to be treated?

Mainly, and often exclusively, by external applications.

Fig. 27.

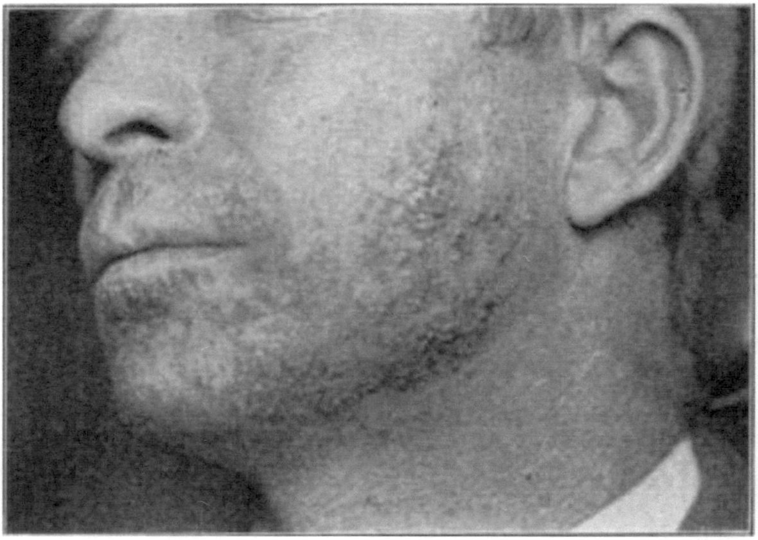

Sycosis.

Is constitutional treatment of no avail in sycosis?

In some instances; but, as a rule, it is negative. If indicated, such remedies as tonics, alteratives, cod-liver oil and the like are to be prescribed.

Describe the external treatment.

Crusting, if present, is to be removed by warm embrocations. If the inflammation is of a high grade, and the parts tender and painful, soothing applications, such as bland oils, black wash and oxide-of-zinc ointment, cold cream and petrolatum, are to be used; [Pg 134] boric-acid solution, fifteen grains to the ounce, may be advised in place of black wash.

In most cases, however, astringent and stimulating remedies are demanded from the start, such as: diachylon ointment, alone or with ten to thirty grains of calomel to the ounce; oleate of mercury, as a five- to twenty-per-cent. ointment; precipitated sulphur, one to three drachms to the ounce of benzoated lard, or lard and lanolin; a ten- to twenty-five-per-cent. ichthyol ointment; and resorcin lotion or ointment, ten to twenty per cent. strength.

Fig. 28.

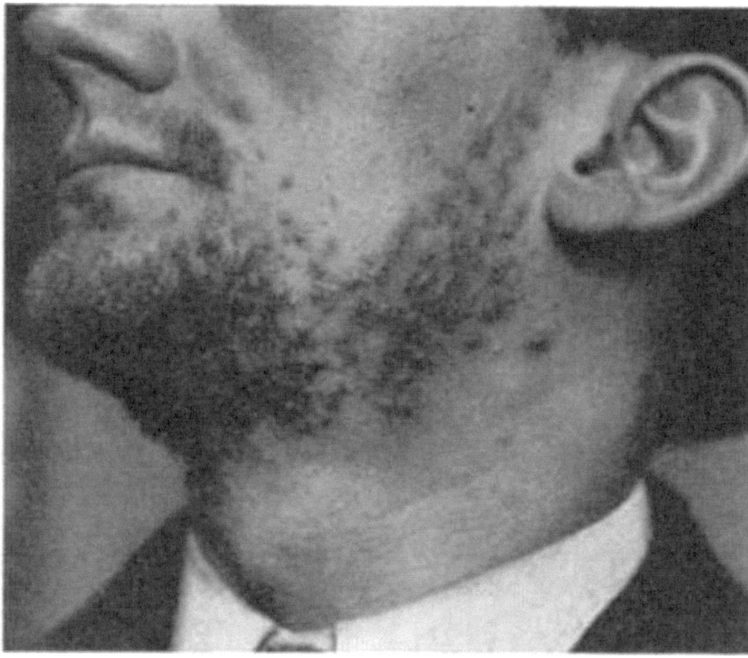

Sycosis.

A change from one application to another will be found necessary in almost all cases.

In obstinate cases the x-ray treatment can be used, as it has proved itself valuable in some instances; as in other diseases, it should be employed cautiously.

What would you advise in regard to shaving?

When bearable (and after a few days' application of soothing remedies it almost always is), it is to be advised in all cases, as it [Pg 135] materially aids in the treatment. After a cure is effected it should be continued for some months, until the healthy condition of the parts is thoroughly established.

When is depilation advisable as a therapeutic measure?

When the suppurative process is active, in order to save the follicles from destruction; incising or puncturing the pustules will often accomplish the same end.

Depilation is in all cases a valuable therapeutic measure, but it is painful; as a routine practice, shaving is less objectionable and, upon the whole, is probably as satisfactory. Those who make free use of the x-ray commonly push it to the point of producing depilation.

Dermatitis Papillaris Capillitii.

(*Synonym:* Acne Keloid.)

Fig. 29.

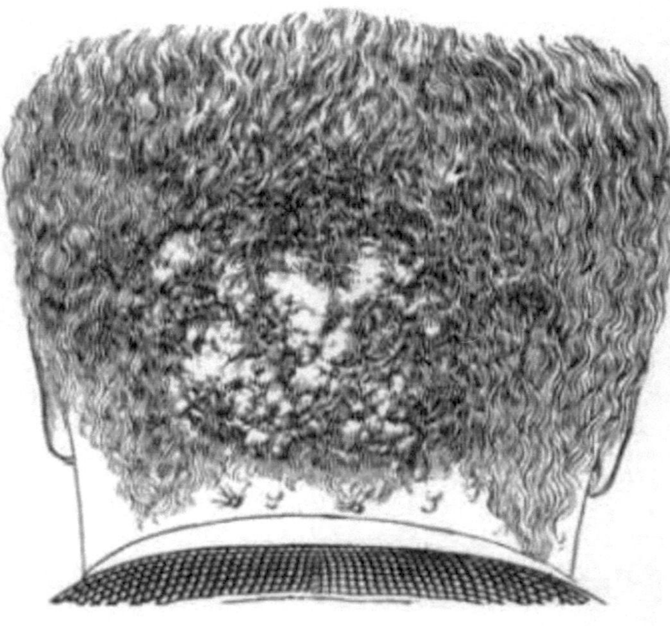

Dermatitis Papillaris Capillitii

Describe dermatitis papillaris capillitii.

This is a peculiar, mildly inflammatory, sycosiform, keloidal, acne-like disease of the hairy border of the back of the neck, often extending upward to the occipital region; partaking, [Pg 136] especially later in its course, somewhat of the nature of keloid. Several or more acne-like lesions, papular and pustular, closely grouped or bunched, appear, developing slowly, usually to the size of peas; are red, pale red, or whitish, often enveloping small tufts of hair, and attended with more or less hair loss. Its course is gradual and persistent. It is an exceedingly rare condition, the exact nature of which is still obscure.

Give the treatment.

Treatment, which is usually unsatisfactory, consists of stimulating applications—the same, in fact, as employed in sycosis, sulphur and ichthyol deserving special mention. Depilation is essential.

Impetigo Contagiosa.

Give a descriptive definition of impetigo contagiosa.

Impetigo contagiosa is an acute, contagious, inflammatory disease, characterized by the formation of discrete, superficial, flat, rounded, or ovalish vesicles or blebs, soon becoming vesicopustular, and drying to thin yellowish crusts.

Upon what parts does the eruption commonly appear?

Upon the face, scalp, and hands, and exceptionally upon other regions.

Describe the symptoms of impetigo contagiosa.

One, several or more small pin-head-sized papulo-vesicles or vesicles make their appearance, usually upon the face and fingers. In the male adult the region of the neck and beard is a favorite situation. They increase in size by extending peripherally, but are more or less flattened and umbilicated, and are without conspicuous areola. The lesions may attain the size of a dime or larger, and when close together may coalesce and form a large patch. In some cases distinct blebs result, and a picture of pemphigus eruption presented; it is probable that many of the cases of "contagious pemphigus" belong to this class. New lesions may appear for several days, but finally, in the course of a week or ten days, they have all dried to thin, wafer-like crusts, of a straw or light-yellow color, but slightly adherent, and appearing as if stuck on; these soon drop off, leaving faint reddish spots, which gradually fade. In some cases there is [Pg 137] so decided a tendency to clear and dry up centrally while spreading peripherally that the eruption has a ring-like aspect; this seems especially so in the bearded region of the male adult.

Instead of presenting as described, it may occur as one or more pea- or finger-nail-sized, rounded and elevated, usually firm, discrete pustules, scattered over one part, or more commonly over various regions, such as the face, hands, feet and lower extremities. The pustules are such from the beginning, and when developed are usually of the size of a pea or finger-nail, elevated, semi-globular or rounded, with somewhat thick and tough walls, and of a whitish or yellowish color; at first there may be a slight inflammatory areola, but as the lesion matures this almost, if not entirely, disappears. The pustules show no disposition to umbilication, rupture or coalescence; drying in the course of several days or a week to yellowish or brownish crusts, which soon drop off, leaving no permanent trace. This variety was formerly thought to be a distinct disease, and was described under the name of *impetigo simplex*.

As a rule there are no constitutional symptoms, but in the more severe cases the eruption may be preceded by febrile disturbance and malaise. Itching may or may not be present.

State the cause of the disease.

It is contagious, the contents of the lesions being inoculable and auto-inoculable. At times it seems to prevail in epidemic form. Pyogenic microörganisms are now regarded as causative. A relationship to vaccination has been alleged by some observers. It is more commonly observed in infants and young children.

From what diseases is impetigo contagiosa to be differentiated?

From eczema, pemphigus, and ecthyma.

How does impetigo contagiosa differ from these several diseases?

By the character of the lesions, their growth, their superficial nature, their course, the absence of an inflammatory base and areola, the thin, yellowish, wafer-like crusts, and usually a history of contagion. [Pg 138]

State the prognosis.

The effect of treatment is usually prompt. The disease, indeed, tends to spontaneous disappearance in two to four weeks; in exceptional instances, more especially in those cases in which itching is present, the excoriations or scratch-marks become inoculated, and in this way it may persist several weeks.

What is the treatment of impetigo contagiosa?

Treatment consists in the destruction of the auto-inoculable properties of the contents of the lesions; this is effected by removing the crusts by means of warm water-and-soap washings, and subsequently rubbing in an ointment of ammoniated mercury, ten to twenty grains to the ounce. Some cases respond more rapidly to the use of a drying ointment, such as Lassar's paste, with ten to twenty grains of white precipitate or sulphur to the ounce. In itching cases, a saturated solution of boric acid, or a carbolic-acid lotion, one to two drachms to the pint, is to be employed for general application.

Impetigo Herpetiformis.

Describe impetigo herpetiformis.

Impetigo herpetiformis is an extremely rare disease, observed usually in pregnant women, and is characterized by the appearance of numerous isolated and closely-crowded pin-head-sized superficial pustules, which show a decided disposition to the formation of circular groups or patches. The central portion of these groups dries to crusts, while new pustules appear at the peripheral portion. They tend to coalesce, and in this manner a greater part of the whole surface may, in the course of weeks or months, become involved. Profound constitutional disturbance, usually of a septic character, precedes and accompanies the disease; in almost every instance a fatal termination sooner or later results.

It is possibly a grave type of dermatitis herpetiformis.

Ecthyma.

Give a descriptive definition of ecthyma.

Ecthyma is a disease characterized by the appearance of one, several or more discrete, finger-nail-sized, flat, usually markedly inflammatory pustules. [Pg 139]

Describe the symptoms and course of ecthyma.

The lesions begin as small, usually pea-sized, pustules; increase somewhat in area, and when fully developed are dime-sized, or larger, somewhat flat, with a markedly inflammatory base and areola. At first yellowish they soon become, from the admixture of blood, reddish, and dry to brownish crusts, beneath which will be found superficial excoriations. The individual pustules are usually somewhat acute in their course, but new lesions may continue to appear from day to day or week to week. As a rule, not more than five to twenty are present at one time, and in most cases they are seated on the legs. More or less pigmentation, and sometimes superficial scarring, may remain to mark the site of the lesions.

Itching is rarely present, but there may be more or less pain and tenderness.

What is the cause of ecthyma?

It is essentially a disease of the poorly cared-for and ill-fed; the direct exciting cause is the introduction of pyogenic microörganisms into the follicular openings. It is closely allied to impetigo contagiosa, and may in fact be regarded as a markedly inflammatory form of the latter affection. It seems much less contagious, however. It is commonly observed in male adults.

From what diseases is ecthyma to be differentiated?

From impetigo contagiosa, and the flat pustular syphiloderm.

How is it distinguished from these several diseases?

The size, shape, inflammatory action, and the depraved general condition, the distribution and lesser-contagiousness will distinguish it from impetigo contagiosa; and the absence of concomitant symptoms of syphilis, and of positive ulceration, as well as its distribution and more rapid and inflammatory course, will exclude the pustular syphiloderm.

State the prognosis.

The disease is readily curable, disappearing upon the removal of the predisposing cause and the employment of local antiseptic applications. [Pg 140]

What treatment is to be advised?

Good food, proper hygiene and tonic remedies; and, locally, removal of the crusts and stimulation of the underlying surface with an ointment of ammoniated mercury, ten to thirty grains to the ounce.

The following mild antiseptic lotion, which materially lessens the tendency to the formation of new lesions, may be applied to the affected region two or three times daily:—

℞ Acidi borici, ... ʒiv Resorcini, ... ʒij Glycerinæ, ... fʒij Alcoholis, ... f℥j Aquæ, ...q.s. ad. .... Oj. M.

A weak lotion of thymol, corrosive sublimate or ichthyol would doubtless be equally effectual.

Pemphigus.

What do you understand by pemphigus?

Pemphigus is an acute or chronic disease characterized by the successive formation of irregularly-scattered, variously-sized blebs.

Name the varieties met with.

Two varieties are usually described—pemphigus vulgaris and pemphigus foliaceus.

Describe the symptoms and course of pemphigus vulgaris.

With or without precursory symptoms of systemic disturbance, irregularly scattered blebs, few or in numbers, make their appearance, arising from erythematous spots or from apparently normal skin. They vary in size from a pea to a large egg, are rounded or ovalish, usually distended, and contain a yellowish fluid which, later, becomes cloudy or puriform. If ruptured, the rete is exposed, but the skin soon regains its normal condition; if undisturbed, the fluid usually disappears by absorption. Each lesion runs its course in several days or a week.

A grave type of pemphigus is exceptionally observed in the new-born—*pemphigus neonatorum.* [Pg 141]

What course does pemphigus vulgaris pursue?

Usually chronic. The disease may subside in several months and the process come to an end, constituting the acute type. As a rule, however, the disease is chronic, new blebs continuing to appear from time to time for an indefinite period.

Fig. 30.

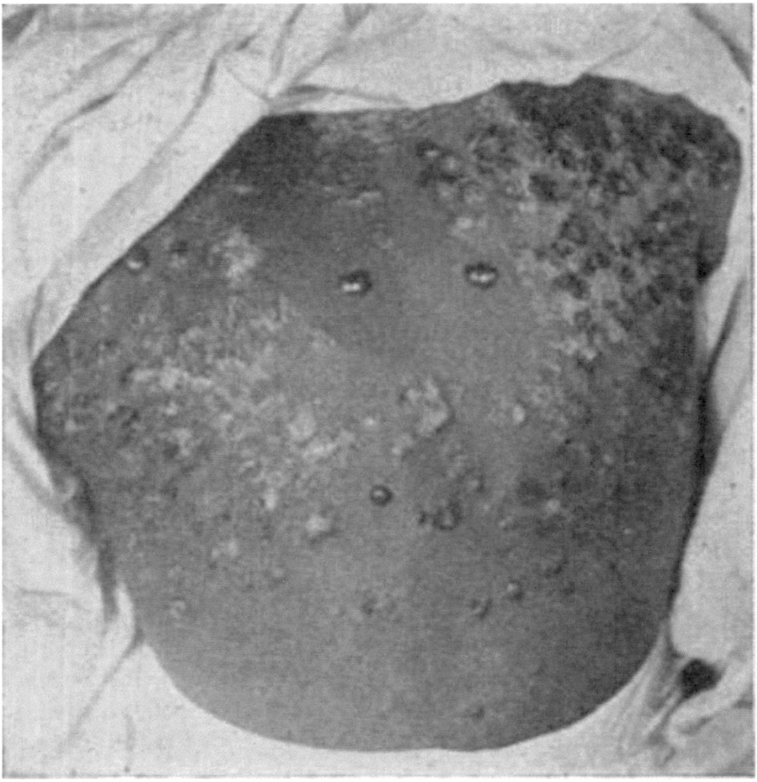

Pemphigus (mulatto).

In what respects does the severe form of pemphigus vulgaris differ from the ordinary type?

In the severe or malignant type the eruption is more profuse; there is marked, and often grave, systemic depression, and the lesions are attended with ulcerative action.

Describe the symptoms and course of pemphigus foliaceus.

In this, the grave type of the disease, the blebs are loose and flaccid, with milky or puriform contents, rupturing and drying to [Pg 142] crusts, which are cast off, disclosing the reddened corium. New blebs appear on the sites of disappearing or half-ruptured lesions, and the whole surface may be thus involved and the disease continue for years, compromising the general health and eventually ending fatally.

In some cases of pemphigus (pemphigus vegetans) a vegetating or papillomatous condition develops from the base of the lesion, with an offensive discharge; it is usually a grave type of the malady.

Exceptionally cases (dermatitis vegetans) are met with which have a close similarity in their symptoms to pemphigus vegetans, but in which the eruption is more or less limited to the genitocrural region. The disorder is not malignant and usually yields to cleanliness and antiseptics.

What is the character of the subjective symptoms in pemphigus?

The subjective symptoms consist variously of heat, tenderness, pain, burning and itching, and may be slight or troublesome.

What is known in regard to the etiology of pemphigus?

The causes are obscure; general debility, overwork, shock, nervous exhaustion, and septic conditions (microörganisms) are thought to be of influence. There seems no doubt that those who have to do with cattle products, especially butchers, are subjects of acute and usually grave pemphigus. Vaccination has exceptionally been responsible for the disease, probably through some coincidental infection. The disease is not contagious, nor is it due to syphilis. It may occur at any age.

It is a rare disease, especially in this country. Most of the cases diagnosed as pemphigus by the inexperienced are examples of bullous urticaria, bullous erythema multiforme, and impetigo contagiosa.

What is the pathology?

The lesions are superficially seated, usually between the horny layer and upper part of the rete. Round-cell infiltration and dilated blood vessels are found about the papillæ and in the subcutaneous tissue. The contents of the blebs, always of alkaline reaction, are [Pg 143] at first serous, later containing blood corpuscles, pus, fatty-acid crystals, epithelial cells, and occasionally uric acid crystals and free ammonia.

From what diseases is pemphigus to be differentiated?

From herpes iris, the bullous syphiloderm, impetigo contagiosa and dermatitis herpetiformis.

How do these several diseases differ from pemphigus?

The acute course, small lesions, concentric arrangement, variegated colors, and distribution, in herpes iris; the thick, bulky, greenish crusts, the underlying ulceration, the course, history, and the presence of concomitant symptoms of syphilis, in the bullous syphiloderm; the history, course, distribution, the character of the crusting, and the contagious and auto-inoculable properties of the contents of the lesions, in impetigo contagiosa; the tendency to appear in groups, the smaller lesions, the intense itchiness, course, multiform characters of the eruption and the disposition to change of type in dermatitis herpetiformis,—will serve as differential points.

State the prognosis of pemphigus.

Its duration is uncertain, and the issue may in severe cases be fatal. In the milder types, after months or several years, recovery may take place.

The extent and severity of the disease and the general condition of the patient are always to be considered before an opinion is expressed.

Pemphigus neonatorum usually ends fatally.

Give the treatment of pemphigus.

Both constitutional and local measures are demanded. Good nutritious food and hygienic regulations are essential. Arsenic and quinia are the most valuable remedies. The former, in occasional instances, seems to have a specific influence, and should always be tried, beginning with small doses and increasing gradually to the point of tolerance and continued for several weeks or longer. The remedy should not be set aside as long as there are signs of improvement, unless the supervention of stomachic, intestinal or other disturbance demand its discontinuance. Other tonics, such as iron, strychnia and cod-liver oil, are also at times of service. [Pg 144] The blebs should be opened and the parts anointed or covered with a mild ointment. In more general cases bran, starch and gelatin baths, and in severe cases the continuous bath, if practicable, are to be used.

CLASS III.—HEMORRHAGES.

Purpura.

Define purpura.

Purpura is a hemorrhagic affection characterized by the appearance of variously-sized, usually non-elevated, smooth, reddish or purplish spots or patches, not disappearing under pressure.

Name the several varieties met with.

Three—purpura simplex, purpura rheumatica and purpura hæmorrhagica; denoting, respectively, the mild, moderate and severe grade of the disease. The division is, to a great extent, an arbitrary one.

Describe the clinical appearance and course of an individual lesion of purpura.

The spot, which may be pin-head, pea-, bean-sized or larger, appears suddenly, and is of a bright red or purplish red color. Its brightness gradually fades, the color changing to a bluish, bluish-green, bluish- or greenish-yellow, dirty yellowish, yellowish-white, and finally disappearing; varying in duration from several days to several weeks.

Describe the symptoms of purpura simplex.

Purpura simplex, or the mild form, shows itself as pin-point to pea- or bean-sized, bright or dark-red spots, limited, as a rule, to the limbs, especially the lower extremities; fading gradually away and coming to an end in a few weeks, or new crops appearing irregularly for several months. There is rarely any systemic disturbance, and, as a rule, no subjective symptoms; in exceptional cases an urticarial element is added—*purpura urticans*.

Describe the symptoms of purpura rheumatica.

Purpura rheumatica (also called *peliosis rheumatica*) is usually preceded by symptoms of malaise, rheumatic pains and sometimes [Pg 145] swelling about the joints; these phenomena abate and frequently disappear upon the outbreak of the eruption. The lesions are pea- to dime-sized, smooth, non-elevated, or slightly raised, and of a reddish or purplish color; the eruption may be more or less generalized, most abundant upon the limbs, or it may be limited to these parts. It may end in a few weeks, or may persist for several months, new spots appearing irregularly or in the form of crops.

As somewhat allied to this is another form (*Schönlein's disease*), quite alarming in its symptoms. It is rare. It is characterized by symptoms partaking of the nature of rheumatism, purpuric spots, blotches and ecchymoses, erythema multiforme, and often associated with considerable edema. The throat is also usually invaded, and indeed the first symptom is commonly in this region. Considerable constitutional disturbance, of a threatening character, is commonly observed. Recovery usually takes place.

Henoch's purpura, observed chiefly in children, resembles the above, with the erythema multiforme character and the œdematous swellings more pronounced, while the actual purpuric symptoms are less conspicuous. Gastric and intestinal symptoms and hemorrhages from the mucous membrane are commonly noted. It is fatal in about 20 per cent. of the cases.

Describe the symptoms of purpura hæmorrhagica.

Purpura hæmorrhagica (also called *land scurvy*) is characterized usually by premonitory, and frequently accompanying, symptoms of general distress, and by the appearance of coin to palm-sized, red or purplish hemorrhagic spots or patches, smooth, non-elevated or raised. Hemorrhage from the mouth, gums and other parts, slight or serious in character, may occur. New lesions continue to appear for several days or weeks; and in exceptional instances, repeated relapses take place, and the disease thus persists for months. It may end fatally.

State the etiology of purpura.

In most instances no cause can be assigned. The disease occurs at all ages from childhood to advanced life, and in individuals, apparently, in good and bad health alike. The hemorrhagic type is oftener seen in subjects debilitated or in a depraved state of health. A microörganism is also looked upon as a factor by some observers, especially in the grave type of disease. [Pg 146]

State the diagnostic characters of purpura.

The appearance, irregularly or in crops, of bright-red or purplish spots, evidently of hemorrhagic nature, and not *disappearing upon pressure*, and as they are fading, going through the several changes of color usually observed in any ecchymosis.

How does scurvy (scorbutus) differ from purpura?

Scurvy, which may resemble the severe grade of purpura, has a different history, a recognizable cause, usually a peculiar distribution, and is accompanied with general weakness and a spongy, soft and bleeding condition of the gums.

What is the pathology of purpura?

The lesion of purpura consists essentially of a hemorrhage into the cutaneous tissues. The blood is subsequently absorbed, the hæmatin undergoing changes of color from a red to greenish and pale yellow, and finally fading away.

State the prognosis

The milder varieties disappear in the course of several weeks or months, and are rarely of serious import; the outcome of purpura hæmorrhagica is somewhat uncertain; although usually favorable, a fatal result from internal hemorrhage is possible. The variety known as Schönlein's disease is alarming, but seldom fatal. Henoch's disease is, however, always of grave import.

What is the treatment of purpura?

Hygienic and dietary measures, the administration of tonics and astringents, and, in severe cases, by relative or absolute rest.

The drugs commonly prescribed are: ergot, oil of erigeron, oil of turpentine, quinia, strychnia, iron, mineral acids, and gallic acid. *External* treatment is rarely called for, but if deemed advisable, astringent lotions may be employed.

Scorbutus.

(*Synonyms:* Scurvy; Sea Scurvy; Purpura Scorbutica.)

Describe scorbutus.

Scurvy is a peculiar constitutional state, developed in those living under bad hygienic conditions, and is characterized by emaciation, [Pg 147] general febrile and asthenic symptoms, a more or less swollen, turgid and spongy and even gangrenous condition of the gums; and concomitantly, or sooner or later, by the appearance, usually upon the lower portion of the legs only, of dark-colored hemorrhagic patches or blotches. The skin of the affected part may become brawny and slightly scaly, and not infrequently may break down and ulcerate. Hemorrhages from the various mucous surfaces, slight or grave, may also take place.

State the etiology of scurvy.

It is due to long-continued deprivation of proper food, especially of fruits and vegetables. Other bad hygienic conditions favor its development. It is seen most commonly in sailors and others taking long voyages.

How is scurvy to be distinguished from purpura?

By the asthenic and emaciated general condition and the peculiar puffy, spongy state of the gums. The cutaneous manifestation is more diffused, forming usually large palm-sized patches, and, as a rule, limited to the region of the ankles or lower part of the legs.

Give the prognosis of scurvy.

The disease is remediable, and usually rapidly so. In those instances in which the same bad hygienic conditions and the ingestion of improper food are continued, death finally results.

What treatment would you advise in scurvy?

Proper food, with an abundance of fruit and vegetables. Lemon or lime juice is especially valuable, and is to be taken freely. If indicated, tonics and stimulants are also to be prescribed. For the relief of the tumid, spongy condition of the gums, astringent and antiseptic mouth washes are to be employed.

The cutaneous manifestations, when tending to ulceration, are to be treated upon general principles. [Pg 148]

CLASS IV.—HYPERTROPHIES.

Lentigo.

(*Synonym:* Freckle.)

Describe lentigo.

Lentigo, or freckle, is characterized by round or irregular, pinhead to pea-sized, yellowish, brownish or blackish spots, occurring usually about the face and the backs of the hands. It is a common affection, varying somewhat in the degree of development; the freckles present may be few and insignificant, or they may exist in profusion and be quite disfiguring. Heat and exposure favor their development. Those of light complexion, especially those with red hair, are its most common subjects. The color of the lesion is usually a yellowish-brown.

It is common to all ages, but is generally seen in its greatest development during adolescence, the disposition to its appearance becoming less marked as age advances.

What is the pathology of lentigo?

Lentigo consists simply of a circumscribed deposit of pigment granules—merely a localized increase of the normal pigment, differing from chloasma (*q. v.*) only in the size and shape of the pigmentation.

State the prognosis.

The blemishes can be removed by treatment, but their return is almost certain.

Name the several applications commonly employed for their removal.

An aqueous or alcoholic solution of corrosive sublimate, one-half to three grains to the ounce; lactic acid, one part to from six to twenty parts of water; and an ointment containing a drachm each of bismuth subnitrate and ammoniated mercury to the ounce.

The applications, which act by removing the epidermal and rete cells and with them the pigment, are made two or three times daily, and their use intermitted for a few days as soon as the skin becomes irritated or scaly.

Touching each freckle for a few seconds with the electric needle, just pricking the epidermis, will occasionally remove the blemish. [Pg 149]

Chloasma.

What do you understand by chloasma?

Chloasma consists of an abnormal deposit of pigment, occurring as variously-sized and shaped, yellowish, brownish or blackish patches.

Describe the clinical appearances of chloasma.

Chloasma appears either in ill-defined patches, as is commonly the case, or as a diffuse discoloration. Its appearance is rapid or gradual, generally the latter. The patches are rounded or irregular, and usually shade off into the sound skin. One, several or more may be present, and coalescence may take place, resulting in a large irregular pigmented area. The color is yellowish, or brownish, and may even be blackish (*melasma, melanoderma*). The skin is otherwise normal. The face is the most common site.

Into what two general classes may the various examples of chloasma be grouped?

Idiopathic and symptomatic.

What cases of chloasma are included in the idiopathic group?

All those cases of pigmentation caused by external agents, such as the sun's rays, sinapisms, blisters, continued cutaneous hyperæmia from scratching or any other cause, etc.

What cases of chloasma are included in the symptomatic group?

All forms of pigment deposit which occur as a consequence of various organic and systemic diseases, as the pigmentation, for instance, seen in association with tuberculosis, cancer, malaria, Addison's disease, uterine affections, and the like. In such cases, with few exceptions, the pigmentation is usually more or less diffuse.

What is chloasma uterinum?

Chloasma uterinum is a term applied to the ill-defined patches of yellowish-brown pigmentation appearing upon the faces of women, usually between the ages of twenty-five and fifty. It is most commonly seen during pregnancy, but may occur in connection with any functional or organic disease of the utero-ovarian apparatus. [Pg 150]

What is argyria?

Argyria is the term applied to the slate-like discoloration which follows the prolonged administration of silver nitrate.

State the pathology of chloasma.

The sole change consists in an increased deposit of pigment.

Give the prognosis of chloasma.

Unless a removal of the exciting or predisposing cause is possible, the prognosis is, as a rule, unfavorable, and the relief furnished by local applications usually but temporary.

If constitutional treatment is advisable, upon what is it to be based?

Upon general principles; there are no special remedies.

How do external remedies act?

Mainly by removing the rete cells and with them the pigmentation; and partly, also, by stimulating the absorbents.

Are all external remedies which tend to remove the upper layers of the skin equally useful for this purpose?

No; on the contrary some such applications are followed by an increase in the pigment deposit.

Name the several applications commonly employed.

Corrosive sublimate in solution, in the strength of one to four grains to the ounce of alcohol and water; a lotion made up as follows:—

> ℞ Hydrargyri chlorid. corros., ... gr. iij-viij Ac. acet. dilut., ... f℥ij Sodii borat., ... ℈ij Aquæ rosæ, ... f℥iv. M.

And also the following:—

> ℞ Hydrargyri chlorid. corros., ... gr. iij-viij Zinci sulphat., Plumbi acetat., ...āā............. ʒss Aquæ, ... f℥iv. M.

And lactic acid, with from five to twenty parts of water; and an [Pg 151] ointment containing a drachm each of bismuth subnitrate and white precipitate to the ounce. Hydrogen peroxide occasionally acts well. Trichloracetic acid, usually weakened with one or two parts water, may be cautiously tried. The application of a strong alcoholic solution of resorcin, twenty to fifty per cent. strength, is also valuable, as is also a two to ten per cent. alcoholic solution of salicylic acid.

(Applications are made two or three times daily, and as soon as slight scaliness or irritation is produced are to be discontinued for one or two days.)

Tattoo-marks are difficult to remove. Excision is the surest method. Electrolysis, applying the needle at various points, somewhat close together, and using a fairly strong current—three to eight milliampères—will exceptionally, especially when repeated several times, produce a reactive inflammation and casting-off of the tissue containing the pigment; a scar is left.

Several writers claim good results with glycerole of papain, pricking it in in the same manner as in tattooing.

Gun-powder marks. If recent, but a day or so after their occurrence, the larger specks may be picked or scraped out. Later, electrolysis, using a fairly strong current, may result in their removal. Their removal may also be satisfactorily effected with a minute cutaneous trephine.

Keratosis Pilaris.

(*Synonyms:* Pityriasis Pilaris; Lichen Pilaris.)

What is meant by keratosis pilaris?

Keratosis pilaris may be defined as a hypertrophic affection characterized by the formation of pin-head-sized, conical, epidermic elevations seated about the apertures of the hair follicles.

Describe the clinical appearances of keratosis pilaris.

The lesions are usually limited to the extensor surfaces of the thighs and arms, especially the former. They appear as pin-head-sized, whitish or grayish elevations, consisting of accumulations of epithelial matter about the apertures of the hair follicles. Each elevation is pierced by a hair, or the hair may be twisted and imprisoned within the epithelial mass; or it may be broken off just at the [Pg 152] point of emergence at the apex of the papule, in which event it may be seen as a dark, central speck. The skin is usually dry, rough and harsh, and in marked cases, to the hand passing over it, feels not unlike a nutmeg-grater. The disease varies in its development, in most cases being so slight as to escape attention. As a rule, it is free from itching.

What course does keratosis pilaris pursue?

It is sluggish and chronic.

Mention some of the etiological factors.

It is not an uncommon disease, and is seen usually in those who are unaccustomed to frequent bathing, being most frequently met with during the winter months. It is chiefly observed during early adult life.

Is there any difficulty in the diagnosis?

No. It is thought at times to bear some resemblance to goose-flesh (cutis anserina), the miliary papular syphiloderm in its desquamating stage, and lichen scrofulosus. In goose-flesh the elevations are evanescent and of an entirely different character; the papules of the syphiloderm are usually generalized, of a reddish color, tend to group, are more solid and deeply-seated, less scaly and are accompanied with other symptoms of syphilis; in lichen scrofulosus the papules are larger, incline to occur in groups, and appear usually upon the abdomen.

State the prognosis.

The disease yields readily to treatment.

Give the treatment of keratosis pilaris.

Frequent warm baths, with the use of a toilet soap or sapo viridis, will usually be found curative. Alkaline baths are also useful. In obstinate cases the ordinary mild ointments, glycerine, etc., are to be advised in conjunction with the baths. [Pg 153]

Keratosis Follicularis.

Describe keratosis follicularis.

Keratosis follicularis (*Darier's disease, ichthyosis follicularis, ichthyosis sebacea cornea, psorospermosis*) is a rare disease characterized by pin-head to pea-sized pointed, rounded, or irregularly-shaped grayish, brownish, red or even black, horny papules or elevations, arising from the sebaceous or hair-follicles. They are, for the most part, discrete, with a tendency here and there to form solid aggregations or areas. Many of them contain projecting cornified plugs which may be squeezed out, leaving pit-like depressions. The face, scalp, lower trunk, groins and flanks are the parts chiefly affected. The view advanced by Darier, that the malady was due to psorosperms, is now denied, the bodies thought to be such having been demonstrated to be due to cell transformation.

As to treatment, in one instance the induction of a substitutive dermatic inflammation had a favorable influence.

Molluscum Epitheliale.

(*Synonyms:* Molluscum Contagiosum; Molluscum Sebaceum; Epithelioma Molluscum.)

Give a definition of molluscum epitheliale.

Molluscum epitheliale is characterized by pin-head to pea-sized, rounded, semi-globular, or flattened, pearl-like elevations, of a whitish or pinkish color.

Describe the symptoms and course of molluscum epitheliale.

The usual seat is the face; not infrequently, however, the growths occur on other parts. The lesions begin as pin-head, waxy-looking, rounded or acuminated elevations, gradually attaining the size of small peas. They have a broad base or occasionally may tend to become pedunculated. They rarely exist in profusion, in most cases three to ten or twelve lesions being present. When fully developed they are somewhat flattened and umbilicated, with a central, darkish point representing the mouth of the follicle. They are whitish or pinkish, and look not unlike drops of wax or pearl buttons. At first they are firm, but eventually, in most cases, tend to become soft and break down. Not infrequently, however, the lesions disappear slowly by absorption, without apparent previous softening. Their course [Pg 154] is usually chronic. The contents, a cheesy-looking mass, may commonly be pressed out without difficulty.

What is the cause of molluscum epitheliale?

It is now generally accepted that the disease is mildly contagious. It occurs chiefly in children, and especially among the poorer classes. The belief in the parasitic nature of the disease is gaining ground; recently the opinion has been advanced that it is due to psorosperms (psorospermosis); but further investigations have indicated that these bodies were degenerated epithelia.

State the pathology.

Fig. 31.

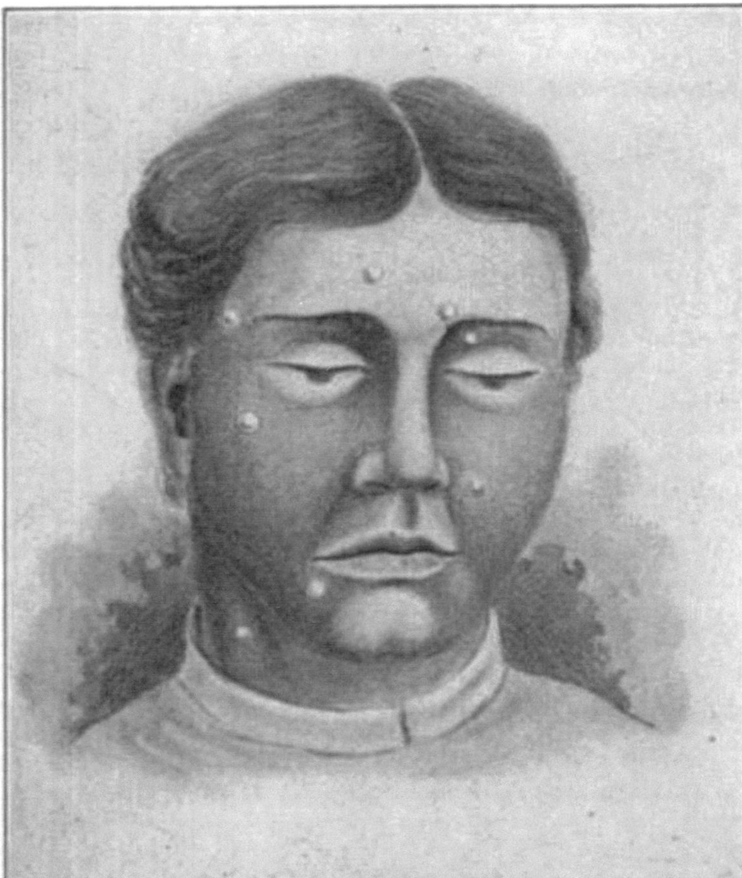

Molluscum Epitheliale.

According to recent investigations, molluscum epitheliale is to be regarded as a hyperplasia of the rete, the growth probably beginning in the hair-follicles; the so-called molluscum bodies—peculiar, [Pg 155] rounded or ovoidal, sharply-defined, fatty-looking bodies found in microscopical examination of the growth—are to be viewed as a form of epithelial degeneration.

What are the diagnostic points in molluscum epitheliale?

The size of the lesions, their waxy or glistening appearance, and the presence of the central orifice.

It is to be differentiated from molluscum fibrosum, warts and acne.

State the prognosis.

The growths are amenable to treatment. In some instances the disease, after existing some weeks, tends to disappear spontaneously.

What is the treatment of molluscum epitheliale?

Incision and expression of the contents, and touching the base of the cavity with silver nitrate. Pedunculated growths may be ligated. In some cases an ointment of ammoniated mercury, twenty to forty grains to the ounce, applied, by gently rubbing, once or twice daily, will bring about a cure.

Callositas.

(*Synonyms:* Tylosis; Tyloma; Callus; Callous; Callosity; Keratoma.)

What do you understand by callositas?

A hard, thickened, horny patch made up of the corneous layers of the epidermis.

Describe the clinical appearances.

Callosities are most common about the hands and feet, and consist of small or large patches of dry, grayish-yellow looking, hard, slight or excessive epidermic accumulations. They are somewhat elevated, especially at the central portion, and gradually merge into the healthy skin. The natural surface lines are in a great measure obliterated, the patches usually being smooth and horn-like.

Keratosis palmaris et plantaris (symmetric keratodermia), as regards the local condition, is a somewhat similar affection. It consists of hypertrophy of the corneous layer of the palm and soles, usually of a more or less horny and plate-like character, but is congenital or hereditary, and not necessarily dependent upon local friction or pressure. [Pg 156]

Are there any inflammatory symptoms in callositas?

No; but exceptionally, from accidental injury, the subjacent corium becomes inflamed, suppurates, and the thickened mass is cast off.

State the causes of callositas.

Pressure and friction; for example, on the hands, from the use of various tools and implements, and on the feet from ill-fitting shoes. It is, indeed, often to be looked upon as an effort of nature to protect the more delicate corium.

In exceptional instances it arises without apparent cause.

What is the pathology?

The epidermis alone is involved; it consists, in fact, of a hyperplasia of the horny layer.

State the prognosis of callositas.

If the causes are removed, the accumulation, as a rule, gradually disappears. The effect of treatment is always rapid and positive, but unless the etiological factors have ceased to act, the result is usually but temporary.

How is callositas treated?

When treatment is deemed advisable, it consists in softening the parts with hot-water soakings or poultices, and subsequently shaving or scraping off the callous mass. The same result may also be often effected by the continuous application, for several days or a week, of a 10 to 15 per cent. salicylated plaster, or the application of a salicylated collodion, same strength; it is followed up by hot-water soaking, the accumulation, as a rule, coming readily away.

Clavus.

(*Synonym:* Corn.)

What is clavus?

Clavus, or corn, is a small, circumscribed, flattened, deep-seated, horny formation usually seated about the toes.

Describe the clinical appearances.

Ordinarily a corn has the appearance of a small callosity; the skin is thickened, polished and horny. Exceptionally, however, [Pg 157] occurring on parts that are naturally more or less moist, as between the toes, maceration takes place, and the result is the so-called *soft corn*. The dorsal aspect of the toes is the common site for the ordinary variety. The usual size is that of a small pea. They are painful on pressure, and, at times, spontaneously so.

State the causes.

Corns are caused by pressure and friction, and may usually be referred to improperly fitting shoes.

What is the pathology of clavus?

It is a hypertrophy of the epiderm. Its shape is conical, with the base external and the apex pressing upon the papillæ. It is, in fact, a peculiarly-shaped callosity, the central portion and apex being dense and horny, forming the so-called core.

Give the treatment of clavus.

A simple method of treatment consists in shaving off, after a preliminary hot-water soaking, the outer portion, and then applying a ring of felt or like material, with the hollow part immediately over the site of the core; this should be worn for several weeks. It is also possible in some cases to extract the whole corn by gently dissecting it out; the after-treatment being the same as the above.

Another method is by means of a ten- to fifteen-per-cent. solution of salicylic acid, in alcohol or collodion, or the following:—

> ℞ Ac. salicylici, ... gr. xxx Ext. cannabis Ind., ... gr. x Collodii, ... fʒiv.
> M.

This is painted on the corn night and morning for several days, at the end of which time the parts are soaked in hot water, and the mass or a greater part of it, will be found, as a rule, to come readily away; one or two repetitions may be necessary. Lactic acid, with one to several parts of water, applied once or twice daily, acts in a similar manner.

Soft corns, after the removal of pressure, may be treated with the solid stick of nitrate of silver, or by any of the methods already mentioned.

In order that treatment be permanently successful, the feet are to be properly fitted. If pressure is removed, corns will commonly disappear spontaneously. [Pg 158]

Cornu Cutaneum.

(*Synonyms:* Cornu Humanum; Cutaneous Horn.)

What is cornu cutaneum?

A cutaneous horn is a circumscribed hypertrophy of the epidermis, forming an outgrowth of horny consistence and of variable size and shape.

At what age and upon what parts are cutaneous horns observed?

They are usually met with late in life, and are mostly seated upon the face and scalp.

Fig. 32.

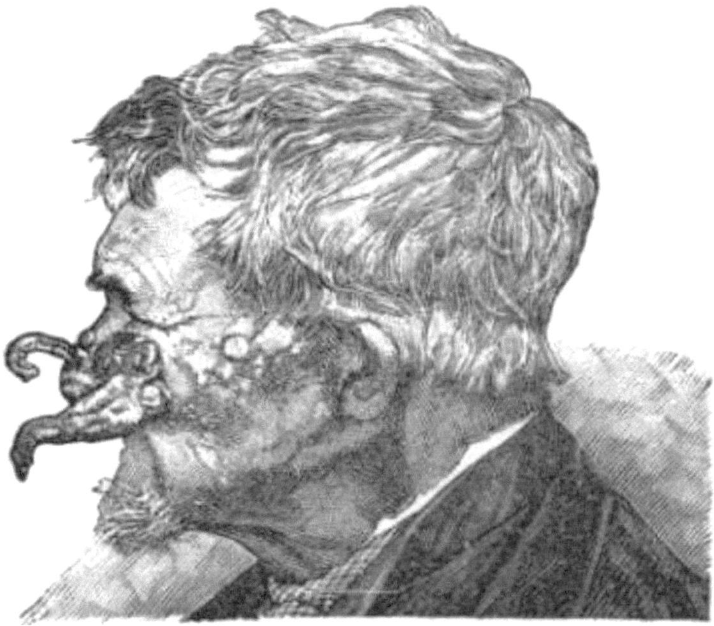

Cutaneous Horns. Showing beginning epitheliomatous degeneration of the base.

(*After Pancoast.*)

Describe the clinical appearances.

In appearance cutaneous horns resemble those seen in the lower animals, differing, if at all, but slightly. They are hard, solid, dry and somewhat brittle; usually tapering, and may be either straight, curved or crooked. Their surface is rough, irregular, laminated or [Pg 159] fissured, the ends pointed, blunt or clubbed. The color varies; it is usually grayish-yellow, but may be even blackish. As commonly seen they are small in size, a fraction of an inch or an inch or thereabouts in length, but exceptionally attain considerable proportions. The base, which rests directly upon the skin, may be broad, flattened, or concave, with the underlying and adjacent tissues normal or the papillæ hypertrophied; and in some cases there is more or less inflammation, which may be followed by suppuration. They are usually solitary formations. They are not, as a rule, painful, unless knocked or irritated.

What course do cutaneous horns pursue?

Their growth is usually slow, and, after having attained a certain size, they not infrequently become loose and fall off; they are almost always reproduced.

What is the cause of these horny growths?

The cause is not known; appearing about the genitalia, they usually develop from acuminated warts. They are rare formations.

State the pathology of cornu cutaneum.

Horns consist of closely agglutinated epidermic cells, forming small columns or rods; in the columns themselves the cells are arranged concentrically. In the base are found hypertrophic papillæ and some bloodvessels. They have their starting-point in the rete mucosum, either from that lying above the papillæ or that lining the follicles and glands.

Does epitheliomatous degeneration of the base ever occur?

Yes.

State the prognosis.

Cutaneous horns may be readily and permanently removed.

What is the treatment?

Treatment consists in detachment, and subsequent destruction of the base; the former is accomplished by dissecting the horn away from the base or forcibly breaking it off, the latter by means of any of the well-known caustics, such as caustic potash, chloride of zinc and the galvano-cautery.

Another method is to excise the base, the horn coming away with it; this necessitates, however, considerable loss of tissue. [Pg 160]

Verruca.

(*Synonym:* Wart.)

What is verruca?

Verruca, or wart, is a hard or soft, rounded, flat, acuminated or filiform, circumscribed epidermal and papillary growth.

Name the several varieties of warts met with.

Verruca vulgaris, verruca plana, verruca plana juvenilis, verruca digitata, verruca filifortnis and verruca acuminata.

Describe verruca vulgaris.

This is the common wart, occurring mostly upon the hands. It is rounded, elevated, circumscribed, hard and horny, with a broad base, and usually the size of a pea. At first it is smooth and covered with slightly thickened epidermis, but later this disappears to some extent, the hypertrophied papillæ, appearing as minute elevations, making up the growth. One, several or more may be present.

Describe verruca plana.

This is the so-called flat wart, and occurs commonly upon the back, especially in elderly people (*verruca senilis, keratosis pigmentosa*). It is, as a rule, but slightly elevated, is usually dark in color, and of the size of a pea or finger-nail.

Describe verruca plana juvenilis.

The warts are mostly pin-head in size, flat, but slightly elevated, rounded, irregular or square-shaped, and of a light yellowish-brown color. They bear resemblance to lichen planus papules. They are apt to be numerous, often becoming aggregated or fused, and occur usually in young children, and, as a rule, on the face and hands.

Describe verruca filiformis.

This is a thread-like growth about an eighth or fourth of an inch long, and occurring commonly about the face, eyelids and neck. It is usually soft to the touch and flexible.

Describe verruca digitata.

This is a variety of wart, which, especially about the edges, is marked by digitations, extending nearly or quite down to the base. It is commonly seen upon the scalp. [Pg 161]

Describe verruca acuminata.

This variety (*venereal wart, pointed wart, pointed condyloma*), usually occurs about the genitalia, especially upon the mucous and mucocutaneous surfaces. It consists of one or more groups of acuminated, pinkish or reddish, raspberry-like elevations, and, according to the region, may be dry or moist; if the latter, the secretion, which is usually yellowish and puriform, from rapid decomposition, develops an offensive and penetrating odor. The formation may be the size of a small pea, or may attain the dimensions of a fist.

What is the cause of warts?

The etiology is not known. They are more common in adolescent and early adult life. Irritating secretions are thought to be causative in the acuminated variety. It is highly probable that a parasitic factor will finally be demonstrated. They are doubtless mildly contagious.

Fig. 33.

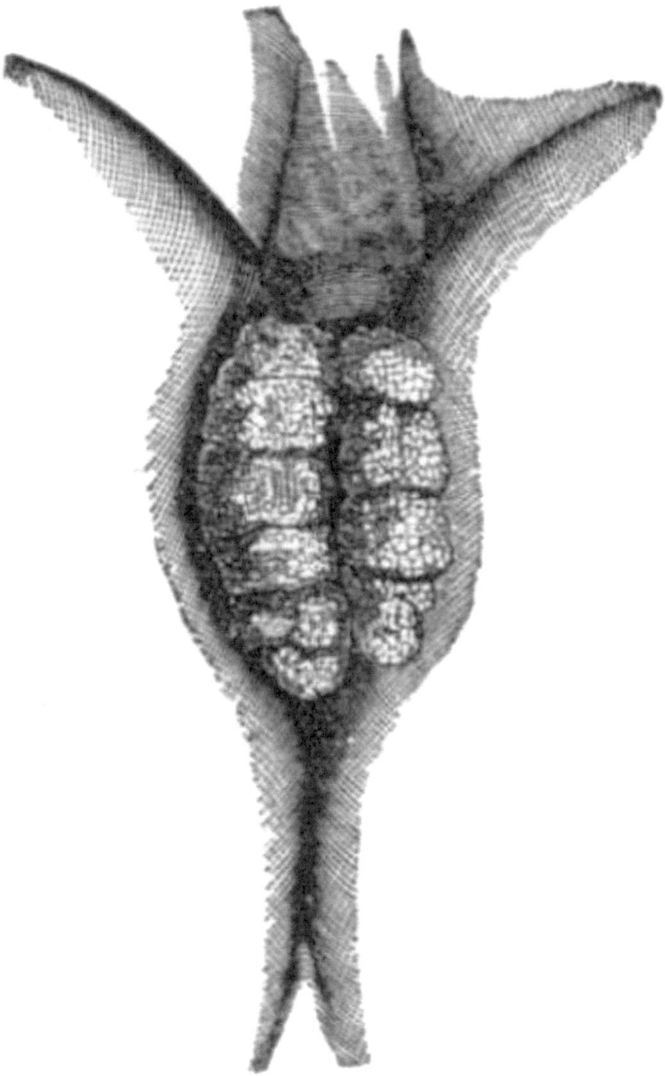

Verruca Acuminata—about the anus. (*After Ashton.*)

State the pathology of warts.

A wart consists of both epidermic and papillary hypertrophy, the interior of the growth containing a vascular loop. In the acuminated variety there are marked papillary enlargement, excessive development of the mucous layer, and an abundant vascular supply. [Pg 162]

Give the treatment of warts.

For ordinary warts, excision or destruction by caustics. The repeated application of a saturated alcoholic solution of salicylic acid is often curative, the upper portion being pared off from time to time. The filiform and digitate varieties may be snipped off with the scissors, and the base touched with nitrate of silver; or a ligature may be used. Curetting is a valuable operative method. The growths may also be removed by electrolysis. When warts are numerous and close together parasiticide applications can be daily made to the whole affected region. For this purpose a boric acid solution, containing five to thirty grains of resorcin to the ounce, and Vleminckx's solution, at first diluted, prove the most valuable.

Verruca acuminata is to be treated by maintaining absolute cleanliness, and the application of such astringents as liquor plumbi subacetatis, tincture of iron, powdered alum and boric acid. The salicylic acid solution may also be used. In obstinate cases, glacial acetic acid or chromic acid may be cautiously employed.

Nævus Pigmentosus.

(*Synonym:* Mole.)

Describe nævus pigmentosus.

Nævus pigmentosus, commonly known as mole, may be defined as a circumscribed increase in the pigment of the skin, usually associated with hypertrophy of one or all of the cutaneous structures, especially of the connective tissue and hair. It occurs singly or in numbers; is usually pea-, bean-sized or larger, rounded or irregular, smooth or rough, flat or elevated, and of a color varying from a light brown to black; the hair found thereon may be either colorless or deeply pigmented, coarse and of considerable length. It is, as a rule, a permanent formation.

Name the several varieties of nævus pigmentosus met with.

Nævus spilus, nævus pilosus, nævus verrucosus, and nævus lipomatodes. So-called linear nævus might also be considered as belonging in this group. [Pg 163]

What is nævus spilus?

A smooth and flat nævus, consisting essentially of augmented pigmentation alone.

Fig. 34.

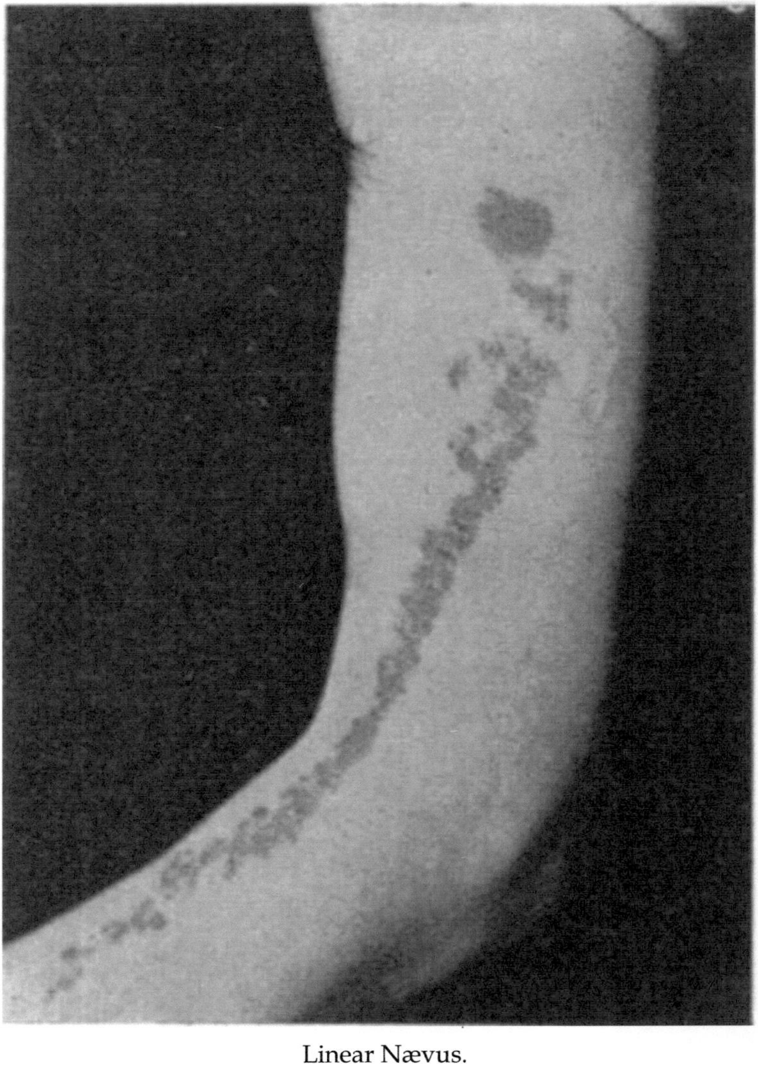

Linear Nævus.

What is nævus pilosus?

A nævus upon which there is an abnormal growth of hair, slight or excessive.

What is nævus verrucosus?

A nævus to which is added hypertrophy of the papillæ, giving rise to a furrowed and uneven surface.

What is linear nævus?

Linear nævus is a formation usually of a verrucous character, more [Pg 164] or less pigmented, sometimes slightly scaly, occurring in band-like or zoster-like areas, and, as a rule, unilaterally.

What is nævus lipomatodes?

A nævus with excessive fat and connective-tissue hypertrophy.

State the etiology of nævus pigmentosus.

The causes are obscure. The growths are usually congenital; but the smooth, non-hairy moles may be acquired.

Give the pathology of nævus pigmentosus.

Microscopical examination shows a marked increase in the pigment in the lowest layers of the rete mucosum, as well as more or less pigmentation in the corium usually following the course of the bloodvessels; in the verrucous variety the papillæ are greatly hypertrophied, in addition to the increased pigmentation. There is, as a rule, more or less connective-tissue hypertrophy.

What is the treatment of nævus pigmentosus?

In many instances interference is scarcely called for, but when demanded consists in the removal of the formation either by the knife, by caustics, or by electrolysis. This last is, in the milder varieties at least, perhaps the best method, as it is less likely to be followed by disfiguring cicatrices. In nævus pilosus the removal of the hairs alone by electrolysis is not infrequently followed by a decided diminution of the pigmentation. In recent years both liquid air and carbon dioxide have also been used successfully in the removal of these growths. Pigmented nævi, which show the least tendency to growth or degenerative change, should be radically removed, as they not infrequently lead to carcinomatous and sarcomatous growths. [Pg 165]

Ichthyosis.

(*Synonym:* Fish-skin Disease.)

Give a descriptive definition of ichthyosis.

Ichthyosis is a chronic, hypertrophic disease, characterized by dryness and scaliness of the skin, with a variable amount of papillary growth.

At what age is ichthyosis first observed?

It is first noticed in infancy or early childhood. In rare instances it is congenital (ichthyosis congenita), and in such cases it is usually severe, and of a grave type; the children are, as a rule, prematurely born, and frequently do not survive many days or weeks.

What extent of surface is involved?

Usually the whole surface, but it is most marked upon the extensor surfaces of the arms and legs, especially at the elbows and knees; the face and scalp, in mild cases, often remain free.

Name the two varieties of ichthyosis usually described.

Ichthyosis simplex and ichthyosis hystrix, terms commonly employed to designate the mild and severe forms respectively.

Describe the clinical appearances of ichthyosis.

The milder forms of the disease may be so slight as to give rise to simple dryness or harshness of the skin (*xeroderma*); but as commonly met with it is more developed, more or less marked scaliness in the form of thin or somewhat thick epidermal plates being present. The papillæ of the skin are often slightly hypertrophied. In slight cases the color of the scales is usually light and pearly; in the more marked examples it is dark gray, olive green or black.

In the severe variety—ichthyosis hystrix—in addition to scaliness there is marked papillary hypertrophy, forming warty or spinous patches. This type is rare, and, as a rule, the surface involved is more or less limited.

Are there any inflammatory symptoms in ichthyosis?

No. In fact, beyond the disfigurement, the disease causes no inconvenience; in those well-marked cases, however, in which the scales are thick and more or less immovable, the natural mobility of the parts is compromised and fissuring often occurs. In the winter [Pg 166] months, in the severer cases, exposed parts may become slightly eczematous.

Does ichthyosis vary somewhat with the season?

Yes. In all cases the disease is better in the warm months, and in the mild forms may entirely disappear during this time. This favorable change is purely mechanical—due to the maceration to which the increased activity of the sweat glands gives rise.

Is the general health affected in ichthyosis?

No.

What course does ichthyosis pursue?

Chronic. Beginning in early infancy or childhood, it usually becomes gradually more marked until adult age, after which time it, as a rule, remains stationary.

What is the etiology?

Beyond a hereditary influence, which is often a positive factor, the causes are obscure. It is not a common disease.

State the pathology.

Anatomically the essential feature is epidermic hypertrophy, with usually a varying degree of papillary hypertrophy also.

Mention the diagnostic features of ichthyosis.

The harsh, dry skin, epidermic and papillary hypertrophy, the furfuraceous or plate-like scaliness, the greater development upon the extensor surfaces, a history of the affection dating from early childhood, and the absence of inflammatory symptoms.

How is ichthyosis to be distinguished from eczema, psoriasis, and other scaly inflammatory diseases?

By the absence of the inflammatory element.

What is the outlook for a case of ichthyosis?

The prognosis is unfavorable as regards a cure, but the process may usually be kept in abeyance or rendered endurable by proper measures.

What treatment would you prescribe for ichthyosis?

Treatment that has in view removal of the scaliness and the maintenance of a soft and flexible condition of the skin. [Pg 167]

In mild cases frequent warm baths, simple or alkaline, will suffice; in others an application of an oily or fatty substance, such as the ordinary oils or ointments, made several hours or immediately before the bath may be necessary. In moderately developed cases the skin is to be washed energetically with sapo viridis and hot water, followed by a warm bath, after which an oily or fatty application is made. In some of the more severe cases the following plan is often useful: The parts are first rubbed with a soapy ointment consisting of one part of precipitated sulphur and seven parts of sapo viridis; a bath is then taken, the skin wiped dry, and a one to five per cent. ointment of salicylic acid gently rubbed in.

Glycerine lotions, one or two drachms to the ounce of water, are also beneficial; as also the following:—

> ℞ Ac. salicylici, ... gr. x-xl Glycerini, ... ʒss-ʒj Lanolin, Petrolati, ...āā ℥ss

In severe cases of ichthyosis hystrix it may be necessary, also, to employ caustics or the knife.

What systemic treatment would you prescribe?

Constitutional remedies are practically powerless; occasionally some good is accomplished by the internal administration of linseed oil and jaborandi.

Onychauxis.

(*Synonym:* Hypertrophy of the Nail.)

Describe onychauxis.

Onychauxis, or hypertrophy of the nail, may take place in one or all directions, and this increase may be, and often is, accompanied by changes in shape, color, and direction of growth. One or all the nails may share in the process. As the result of lateral deviation of growth, the nail presses upon the surrounding tissues, producing a varying degree of inflammation—*paronychia.*

What is the etiology of hypertrophy of the nail?

The condition may be either congenital or acquired. In the latter [Pg 168] instances it is usually the result of the extension to the matrix of such cutaneous diseases as psoriasis and eczema; or it is produced by constitutional maladies, such as syphilis.

Give the treatment of hypertrophy of the nail.

Treatment consists in the removal of the redundant nail-tissue by means of the knife or scissors; and, when dependent upon eczema or psoriasis, the employment of remedies suitable for these diseases. When it is the result of syphilis, the medication appropriate to this disease is to be employed.

In paronychia the nail should be frequently trimmed and a pledget of lint or cotton be interposed between the edge of the nail and the adjacent soft parts; astringent powders and lotions may often be employed with advantage; and in severe and persistent cases excision of the nail, partial or complete, may be found necessary.

Hypertrichosis.

(*Synonyms:* Hirsuties; Hypertrophy of the Hair; Superfluous Hair.)

What is meant by hypertrichosis?

Hypertrichosis is a term applied to excessive growth of hair, either as regards region, extent, age or sex.

Describe the several conditions met with.

The unnatural hair growth may be slight, as, for instance, upon a nævus (*nævus pilosus*); or it may be excessive, as in the so-called hairy people (*homines pilosi*); or it may also appear on the face, arms and other parts in females, resulting from a hypertrophy of the natural lanugo hairs.

State the causes of hypertrichosis.

Hereditary influence is often a factor; the condition may also be congenital.

If acquired, the tendency manifests itself usually toward middle life. In women, it is not infrequently associated with diseases of the utero-ovarian system; in many instances, however, there is no apparent cause. Local irritation or stimulation has at times a causative influence. [Pg 169]

How is hypertrichosis to be treated?

For general hypertrichosis there is no remedy. Small hairy nævi may be excised, or, as also in the larger hairy moles, the hairs may be removed by electrolysis.

On the faces of women, if the hairs are coarse or large, electrolysis constitutes the only satisfactory method; if the hairs are small and lanugo-like, the operation is not to be advised. It is somewhat painful, but never unbearable. In the past several years the *x*-ray has been advocated by several writers, but it requires usually numerous exposures pushed to the point of producing erythema; it is not without risk, and the hairs are said to return in some months.

What temporary methods are usually resorted to for the removal of superfluous hair?

Shaving, extraction of the hairs and the use of depilatories. As a depilatory, a powder made up of two drachms of barium sulphide and three drachms each of zinc oxide and starch, is commonly (and cautiously) employed; at the time of application enough water is added to the powder to make a paste, and it is then spread thinly upon the parts, allowed to remain five to fifteen minutes, or until heat of skin or a burning sensation is felt, washed off thoroughly, and a soothing ointment applied. This preparation must be well prepared to be efficient.

Describe the method of removal of superfluous hair by electrolysis.

A fine needle in a suitable handle is attached to the *negative* pole of a *galvanic* battery, introduced into the hair-follicle to the depth of the papilla, and the circuit completed by the patient touching the positive electrode; in several seconds slight blanching and frothing usually appear at the point of insertion; a few seconds later the current is broken by release of the positive electrode, and the needle is then withdrawn. Sometimes a wheal-like elevation arises, remains several minutes or hours, and then disappears; or occasionally, probably from secondary infection, it develops into a pustule.

A strength of current of a half to two milliamperes is usually sufficient; the time necessary for the destruction of the papilla varying from several to thirty seconds. [Pg 170]

How are you to know if the papilla has been destroyed?

The hair will readily come out with but little, if any, traction.

What is the result if the current has been too strong or too long continued?

The follicle suppurates and a scar results.

Why should contiguous hairs not be operated upon at the same sitting?

In order that the chances of marked inflammatory action and scarring (always possibilities) may be reduced to a minimum.

In case of failure to destroy an individual papilla, should a second attempt be made at the same sitting?

As a rule not, in order to avoid the possibility of too much destructive action, and consequent scarring.

Can scarring always be prevented?

In the average case, with skill and care, the use of an exceedingly fine needle and the avoidance of too strong a current, *perceptible* scarring (scarring perceptible to the ordinary observer or at ordinary distance) need rarely occur.

What measures are to be advised for the irritation produced by the operation?

Hot-water applications and the use of an ointment made of two drachms cold cream and ten grains of boric acid are of advantage not only in reducing the resulting hyperæmia, but also in preventing suppuration and consequent scarring. To lessen the chances of the latter, cleansing the parts with alcohol just before and after the operation is also of service.

Œdema Neonatorum.

Describe œdema neonatorum.

The essential symptoms are œdema and a variable degree of hardness and induration. It develops in the first few days of life, and usually upon the extremities, especially the lower. It may remain more or less limited to these parts, but, as a rule, slowly extends. [Pg 171] The skin is of a yellowish, dusky, or livid color, and sometimes glossy or shining. There are general symptoms of drowsiness, subnormal temperature, weakened circulation, and impaired respiration, which gradually increase, and in eighty to ninety per cent. of the cases lead to death. It is believed to be similar to anasarca in the adult and to be due to like causes.

Treatment consists in maintaining the body-heat, sufficient and proper nourishment and stimulation.

Sclerema Neonatorum.

(*Synonyms:* Scleroderma Neonatorum; Sclerema of the Newborn.)

What is sclerema neonatorum?

Sclerema neonatorum is a disease of infancy, showing itself usually at or shortly after birth, and is characterized by a diffuse stiffness and rigidity of the integument, accompanied by coldness, œdema, discoloration, lividity and general circulatory disturbance.

Describe the symptoms, course, nature and treatment of sclerema neonatorum.

As a rule the disease first manifests itself upon the lower extremities, and then gradually, but usually rapidly, invades the trunk, arms and face. The surface is cold. The skin, which is noted to be reddish, purplish or mottled, is œdematous, stiff and tense; in consequence the infant is unable to move, respires feebly and usually perishes in a few days or weeks. In extremely exceptional instances the disease, after involving a small part, may retrogress and recovery take place.

The disease is rare, and in most cases is found associated with pneumonia and with affections of the circulatory apparatus.

Treatment should be directed toward maintaining warmth and proper alimentation. [Pg 172]

Scleroderma.

(*Synonyms:* Sclerema; Scleriasis; Dermatosclerosis; Morphœa; Keloid of Addison.)

What is scleroderma?

Scleroderma is an acute or chronic disease of the skin characterized by a localized or general, more or less diffuse, usually pigmented, rigid, stiffened, indurated or hide-bound condition.

Morphœa, by some formerly thought to be a distinct affection, is now believed to be a form of scleroderma; as typically met with it is characterized by one or more rounded, oval, or elongate, coin- to palm-sized, pinkish, or whitish ivory-looking patches. In some instances such patches are seen in association with the more classic type of scleroderma just defined.

Describe the symptoms of ordinary scleroderma.

The disease may be acute or chronic, usually the latter. A portion or almost the entire surface may be involved, or it may occupy variously sized and shaped areas. The integument becomes more or less rigid and indurated, hard to the touch, hide-bound, and in marked cases immobile. Œdema may, especially in the more acute cases, precede the induration. Pigmentation, of a yellowish or brownish color, is often a precursory and accompanying symptom. The skin feels tight and contracted, and in some instances numbness and cramp-like pains are complained of.

Describe the variety known as morphœa.

The patches (one, several, or more), occurring most frequently about the trunk, are in the beginning usually slightly hyperæmic, later becoming pale-yellowish or white, and having a pinkish or lilac border made up of minute capillaries. They are, as a rule, sharply defined, with a smooth, often shining and atrophic-looking surface; are soft, fine or leathery to the touch, on a level or somewhat depressed, and appearing not unlike a piece of bacon or ivory laid in the skin. Occasionally the patches are noted to occur over nerve-tracts. The adjacent skin may be normal or there may be more or [Pg 173] less yellowish or brownish mottling. The subjective symptoms of tingling, itching, numbness, and even pain, may or may not be present.

What is the course of the disease?

Sooner or later, usually after months or years, the disease ends in resolution and recovery, or in marked atrophic changes, causing contraction and deformity. As a rule, the general health remains good.

State the causes of scleroderma.

The condition is to be considered as probably of neurotic origin. Exposure and shock to the nervous system are to be looked upon as influential. It is a rare disease, observed usually in early adult or middle life, and is more frequent in women than in men.

What is the pathology?

In typical and advanced cases both the true skin and the subcutaneous connective tissue show a marked increase of connective tissue-element, with thickening and condensation of the fibers.

Is there any difficulty in reaching a diagnosis in scleroderma?

As a rule, no. The characters—rigidity, stiffness, hardness, and hide-bound condition of the skin—are always distinctive.

The peculiar appearance, the course and character of the patches, of morphœa are quite distinctive.

Give the prognosis of scleroderma.

It should always be guarded. In many instances recovery takes place, whilst in others the disease is rebellious, lasting indefinitely. The prognosis of the variety known as morphœa is less unfavorable than general scleroderma, and recovery more frequent.

What is the treatment of scleroderma?

Tonics, such as arsenic, quinia, nux vomica, and cod-liver oil; conjointly with the local employment of stimulating, oily or fatty applications, friction, and electricity. Röntgen-ray treatment is often of value, more especially in the morphœa type. [Pg 174]

Elephantiasis.

(*Synonyms:* Elephantiasis Arabum; Pachydermia; Barbadoes Leg; Elephant Leg.)

Give a descriptive definition of elephantiasis.

Elephantiasis is a chronic hypertrophic disease of the skin and subcutaneous tissue characterized by enlargement and deformity, lymphangitis, swelling, œdema, thickening, induration, pigmentation, and more or less papillary growth.

Fig. 35.

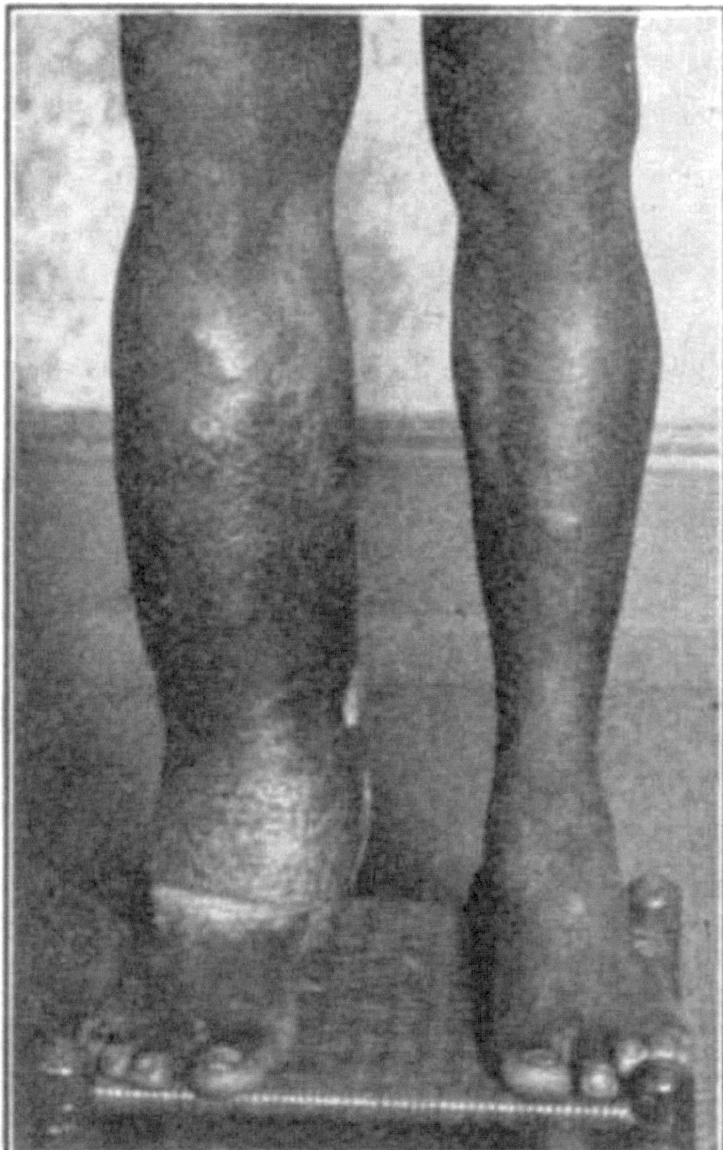

Elephantiasis of moderate development.

What parts are commonly involved in elephantiasis?

Usually one or both legs; occasionally the genitalia; other parts are seldom affected.

Describe the symptoms of elephantiasis.

The disease usually begins with recurrent (at intervals of months or years) erysipelatous inflammation, with swelling, pain, heat, redness and lymphangitis; after each attack the parts remain somewhat [Pg 175] increased in size, although at first not noticeably so. After months or one or two years the enlargement or hypertrophy becomes conspicuous, the part is chronically swollen, œdematous and hard; the skin is thickened, the normal lines and folds exaggerated, the papillæ enlarged and prominent, and with more or less fissuring and pigmentation.

What is the further course of the disease?

There is gradual increase in size, the parts in some instances reaching enormous proportions; the skin becomes rough and warty, eczematous inflammation is often superadded, and, sooner or later, ulcers, superficial or deep, form—which, together with the crusting and moderate scaliness, present a striking picture. There may be periods of comparative inactivity, or, after reaching a certain development, the disease may, for a time at least, remain stationary.

Are there any subjective symptoms?

A variable degree of pain is often noted, especially marked during the inflammatory attacks. The general health is not involved.

State the cause of elephantiasis.

The etiology is obscure. The disease rarely occurs before puberty. It is most common in tropical countries, more especially among the poor and neglected. It is not hereditary, nor can it be said to be contagious. Inflammation and obstruction of the lymphatics, probably due, according to late investigations, to the presence of large numbers of filaria (microscopic thread-worms) in the lymph channels and bloodvessels, is to be looked upon as the immediate cause.

What is the pathology?

All parts of the skin and subcutaneous connective-tissue are hypertrophied, the lymphatic glands are swollen, the lymph channels and bloodvessels enlarged, and there is more or less inflammation, with œdema. Secondarily, from pressure, atrophy and destruction of the skin-glands, and atrophic degeneration of the fat and muscles result.

What are the diagnostic characters of beginning elephantiasis?

Recurrent erysipelatous inflammation, attended with gradual enlargement of the parts. [Pg 176]

The appearances, later in the course of the disease, are so characteristic that a mistake is scarcely possible.

Give the prognosis of elephantiasis.

If the case comes under treatment in the first months of its development, the process may probably be checked or held in abeyance; when well established, rarely more than palliation is possible.

What is the treatment of elephantiasis?

The inflammatory attacks are to be treated on general principles. Quinia, potassium iodide, iron and other tonics are occasionally useful; and, especially in the earlier stages, climatic change is often of value. Between the inflammatory attacks the parts are to be rubbed with an ointment of iodine or mercury, together with galvanization of the involved part.

In elephantiasis of the leg, a roller or rubber bandage, or the gum stocking, is to be worn; compression and ligation of the main artery, and even excision of the sciatic nerve, have all been employed, with more or less diminution in size as a result. In elephantiasis of the genitalia, if the disease is well advanced, excision or amputation of the parts is to be practised.

Eczematous inflammation, if present, is to be treated with the ordinary remedies.

Dermatolysis.

(*Synonym:* Cutis Pendula.)

Give a descriptive definition of dermatolysis.

Dermatolysis is a rare disease, consisting of hypertrophy and looseness of the skin and subcutaneous connective tissue, with a tendency to hang in folds.

Describe the symptoms and course of dermatolysis.

It may be congenital or acquired, and maybe limited to a small or large area, or develop simultaneously at several regions. All parts of the skin, including the follicles, glands and subcutaneous connective and areolar tissue, share in the hypertrophy; and this in exceptional instances may be so extensive that the integument hangs in folds. The enlargement of the follicles, natural folds and rugæ gives rise to an uneven surface, but the skin remains soft and [Pg 177] pliable. There is also increased pigmentation, the integument becoming more or less brownish.

What course does dermatolysis pursue?

Its development is slow and usually progressive. It gives rise to no further inconvenience than its weight and consequent discomfort.

Give the etiology.

The etiology is obscure. It is considered by some authors as allied to molluscum fibrosum, and, in fact, as a manifestation of that disease, ordinary molluscum tumors sometimes being associated with it. It is not malignant.

What is the pathology?

The disease consists of a simple hypertrophy of all the skin structures and the subcutaneous connective tissue.

What is the treatment of dermatolysis?

Excision when advisable and practicable.

CLASS V.—ATROPHIES.

Albinismus.

What do you understand by albinismus?

Congenital absence, either partial or complete, of the pigment normally present in the skin, hair and eyes.

Describe complete albinismus.

In complete albinismus the skin of the entire body is white, the hair very fine, soft and white or whitish-yellow in color, the irides are colorless or light blue, and the pupils, owing to the absence of pigment in the choroid, are red; this absence of pigment in the eyes gives rise to photophobia and nystagmus. *Albinos*—a term applied to such individuals—are commonly of feeble constitution, and may exhibit imperfect mental development.

Describe partial albinismus.

Partial albinismus is met with most frequently in the colored race. In this form of the affection the pigment is absent in one, several or [Pg 178] more variously-sized patches; usually the hairs growing thereon are likewise colorless.

Is there any structural change in the skin?

No. The functions of the skin are performed in a perfectly natural manner, and microscopical examination shows no departure from normal structure save the complete absence of pigment.

What is known in regard to the etiology?

Nothing is known of the causes producing albinismus beyond the single fact that it is frequently hereditary.

Does albinismus admit of treatment?

No; the condition is without remedy.

Vitiligo.

(*Synonyms:* Leucoderma; Leucopathia.)

Give a definition of vitiligo.

Vitiligo may be defined as a disease involving the pigment of the skin alone, characterized by several or more progressive, milky-white patches surrounded by increased pigmentation.

Describe the symptoms of vitiligo.

The disease may begin at one or more regions, the backs of the hands, trunk and face being favorite parts; its appearance is usually insidious, and the spots may not be especially noticeable until they are the size of a pea or larger. The patches grow slowly, are milky or dead white, smooth, non-elevated, and of rounded outline; the bordering skin is darker than normal, showing increased pigmentation. Several contiguous spots may coalesce and form a large, irregularly-shaped patch. Hair growing on the involved skin may or may not be blanched.

There are no subjective symptoms.

What course does vitiligo pursue?

The course of the disease is slow, months and sometimes years elapsing before it reaches conspicuous development. It may after a time remain stationary, or, in rare instances, retrogress; as a rule, however, it is progressive. Exceptionally, the greater part, or even the whole surface may eventually be involved. [Pg 179]

Give the etiology of vitiligo.

Disturbed innervation is thought to be influential. The disease develops often without apparent cause. Alopecia areata and morphœa have been observed associated with it.

Fig. 36.

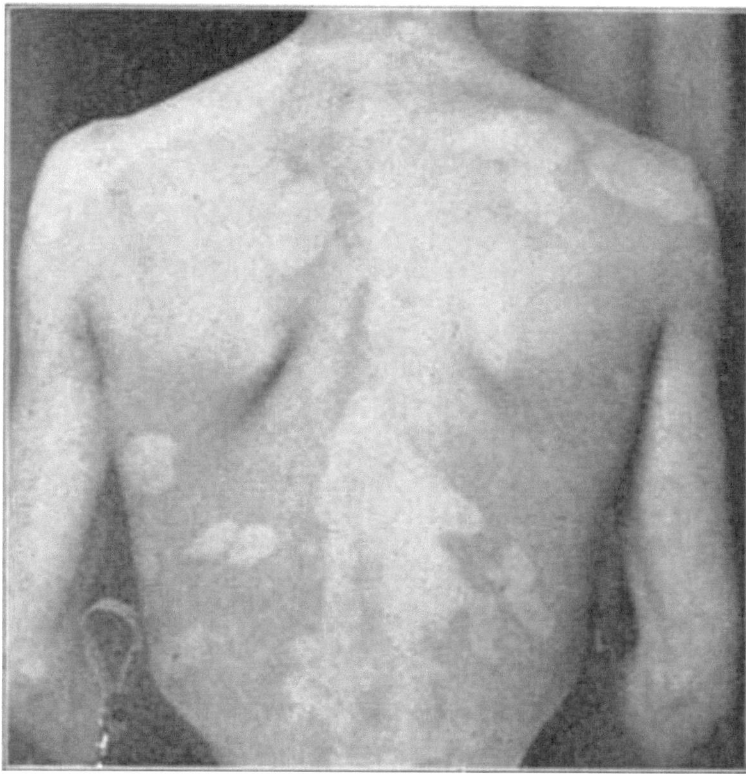

Vitiligo.

State the pathology of vitiligo.

The disease consists, anatomically, of both a diminution and increase of the pigment—the white patch resulting from the former, and the pigmented borders from the latter. There is no textural change, the skin in other respects being normal.

From what diseases is vitiligo to be differentiated?

From morphœa and from the anæsthetic patches of leprosy.

In what respects do these diseases differ from vitiligo?

In morphœa there is textural change, and in leprosy both textural change and constitutional or other symptoms. [Pg 180]

What prognosis is to be given?

It should always be guarded, the disease in almost all cases being irresponsive to treatment.

What is the treatment of vitiligo?

The general health is to be looked after, and remedies directed especially toward the nervous system to be employed. Arsenic, in small and continued doses, seems at times to have an influence; when there is lack of general tone it may be prescribed as follows:—

> ℞ Liq. potassii arsenitis, ... fʒj Tinct. nucis vom., ... fʒiij Elix. calisayæ, ... q.s. ad. .... f℥iv. M. SIG.—fʒj t.d.

Suprarenal-gland preparations in moderate dosage long continued has appeared in a few instances to be of some benefit.

When upon exposed parts, stimulation of the patches, with the view of producing hyperæmia and consequent pigment deposit; conjoined with suitable applications to the surrounding pigmented skin, with a view to lessen the coloration (see *treatment of chloasma*), will be of aid in rendering the disease less conspicuous. Or the condition may be, in a measure, masked by staining the patches with walnut juice or similar pigment.

Canities.

(*Synonym:* Grayness of the Hair.)

Describe canities.

Canities, or graying of the hair, may occur in localized areas or it may be more or less general; the blanching may be slight, scarcely amounting to slight grayness, or it may be complete. It is common to advancing years (*canities senilis*); it is seen also exceptionally in early life (*canities præmatura*). The condition is usually permanent. The loss of pigment takes place, as a rule, slowly, but several apparently authentic cases have been reported in which the change occurred in the course of a night or in a few days.

What is the etiology of canities?

The causes are obscure. Heredity is usually an influential factor, [Pg 181] and conditions which impair the general nutrition have at times an etiological bearing. Intense anxiety, fright, and other profound nervous shock are looked upon as causative in sudden graying of the hair.

Give the treatment.

Canities is without remedy. Dyeing, although not to be advised, is often practised, and the condition thus masked.

Alopecia.

(*Synonym:* Baldness.)

What do you understand by alopecia?

By alopecia is meant loss of hair, either partial or complete.

Name the several varieties of alopecia.

The so-called varieties are based mainly upon the etiology, and are named congenital alopecia, premature alopecia and senile alopecia.

Describe congenital alopecia.

Congenital alopecia is a rare condition, in which the hair-loss is usually noted to be patchy, or the general hair-growth may simply be scanty. In rare instances the hair has been entirely wanting; in such cases there is usually defective development of other structures, such as the teeth.

Describe premature alopecia.

Loss of hair occurring in early and middle adult life is not uncommon, and may consist of a simple thinning or of more or less complete baldness of the whole or greater part of the scalp. It usually develops slowly, some months or several years passing before the condition is well established. It is often idiopathic, and without apparent cause further than probably a hereditary predisposition. It may also be symptomatic, as, for example, the loss of hair, usually rapid (*defluvium capillorum*), following systemic diseases, such as the various fevers, and syphilis; or as a result of a long-continued seborrhœa or seborrhœic eczema (*alopecia furfuracea*).

Describe senile alopecia.

This is the baldness so frequently seen developing with advancing years, and may consist merely of a general thinning, or, more [Pg 182] commonly, a general thinning with a more or less complete baldness of the temporal and anterior portion or of the vertex of the scalp.

What is the prognosis in the various varieties of alopecia?

In those cases in which there is a positive cause, as, for instance, in symptomatic alopecia, the prognosis is, as a rule, favorable, especially if no family predisposition exists. In the congenital and senile varieties the condition is usually irremediable. In idiopathic premature alopecia, the prognosis should be extremely guarded.

How would you treat alopecia?

By removing or modifying the predisposing factors by appropriate constitutional remedies, and by the external use of stimulating applications.

Name several remedies or combinations usually employed in the local treatment.

Sulphur ointment, full strength or weakened with lard or vaseline; a lotion of resorcin consisting of one or two drachms to four ounces of alcohol, to which is added ten to thirty minims of castor oil; and a lotion made up as follows:—

> ℞ Tinct. cantharidis, ... fʒiv Tinct. capsici, ... f℥j Ol. ricini, ... fʒss-fʒj Alcoholis, ... q.s. ad. .... f℥iv. M.

The following is sometimes beneficial:—

> ℞ Resorcin, ... gr. lxxx Quininæ (alkaloid), ... gr. xv Ol. ricini, ... ♏v-♏xx Alcoholis, ... f℥iv. M.

Another excellent formula is:

> ℞ Resorcin, ... gr. lxxx-cxx Ac. carbolici cryst., ... gr. xx Spts. myrciæ, ... f℥iv. M.

And also the various other stimulating applications employed in alopecia areata (*q. v.*). [Pg 183]

Other measures of value are: Faradic electricity applied daily for five minutes with a metallic brush or comb; daily massage, with the object of loosening the skin and giving more freedom to cutaneous and subcutaneous circulation; and the application, two or three times weekly, of static electricity by means of the static crown electrode.

(The application selected should be gently—not rubbing—applied daily or every second or third day, according to the case; if a lotion, moistening the parts with it; if an ointment, merely greasing the parts. Shampooing every one to three weeks, according to circumstances.)

Alopecia Areata.

(*Synonyms:* Area Celsi; Alopecia Circumscripta.)

What do you understand by alopecia areata?

Fig. 37.

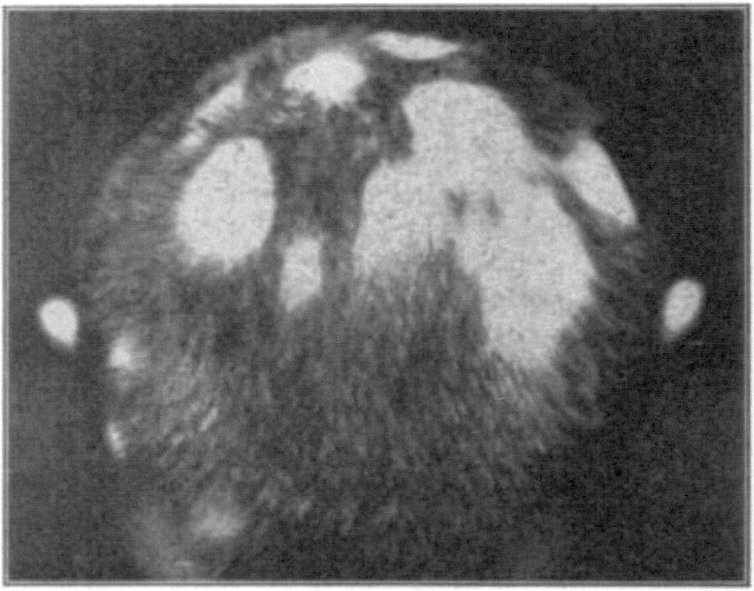

Alopecia Areata.

Alopecia areata is an affection of the hairy system, in which occur one or more circumscribed, round or oval patches of complete baldness unattended by any marked alteration in the skin. [Pg 184]

Upon what parts and at what age does the disease occur?

In the large majority of cases the disease is limited to the scalp; but it may invade other portions of the body, as the bearded region, eyebrows, eyelashes, and, in rare instances, the entire integument.

It is most common between the ages of ten and forty.

Describe the symptoms of alopecia areata.

The disease begins either suddenly, without premonitory symptoms, one or several patches being formed in a few hours; or, and as is more usually the case, several days or weeks elapse before the bald area or areas are sufficiently large to become noticeable. The patches continue to extend peripherally for a variable period, and then remain stationary, or several gradually coalesce and form a large, irregular area involving the entire or a greater portion of the scalp. The skin of the affected regions is smooth, faintly pink or milky white,

Fig. 38.

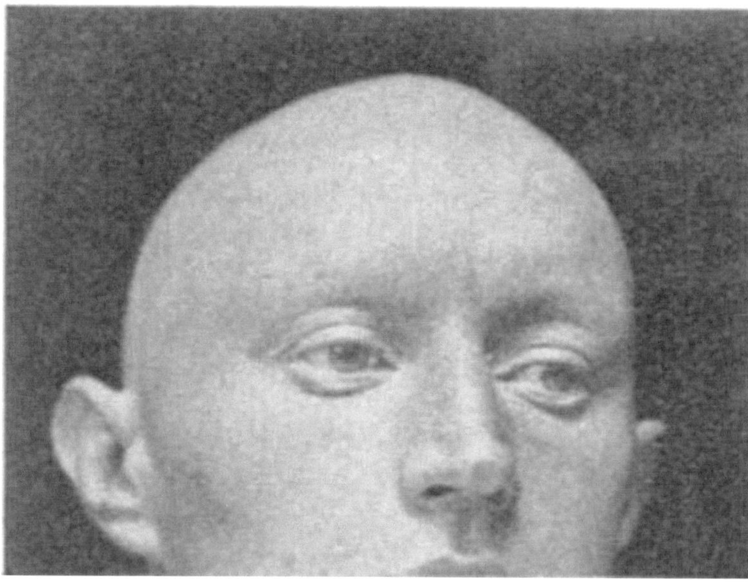

Alopecia Areata—complete hair loss.

and at first presents no departure from the normal; sooner or later, however, the follicles become less prominent, and slight atrophy or thinning may occur, the bald plaques being slightly depressed.

Occasionally, usually about the periphery and in the early stages, a few hair-stumps may be seen. [Pg 185]

What course does alopecia areata pursue?

Almost invariably chronic. After the lapse of a variable period the patches cease to extend, the hairs at the margins of the bald areas being firmly fixed in the follicles; sooner or later a fine, colorless lanugo or down shows itself, which may continue to grow until it is about a half-inch or so in length and then drop out; or it may remain, become coarser and pigmented, and the parts resume their normal condition. Not infrequently, however, after growing for a time, the new hair falls out, and this may happen several times before the termination of the disease.

Are there any subjective symptoms in alopecia areata?

As a rule, not; but occasionally the appearance of the patches is preceded by severe headache, itching or burning, or other manifestations of disturbed innervation.

State the cause of alopecia areata.

The etiology is obscure. Two theories as to the cause of the disease exist: one of these regards it as parasitic, and the other considers it to be trophoneurotic. Doubtless both are right, as a study of the literature would indicate that there are, as regards etiology, really two varieties—the contagious and the non-contagious. In America examples of the contagious variety are uncommon.

Does the skin undergo any alterative or destructive changes?

Microscopical examination of the skin of the diseased area shows little or no alteration in its structure beyond slight thinning.

How do you distinguish alopecia areata from ringworm?

The plaques of alopecia areata are smooth, often completely devoid of hair, and free from scales; while those of ringworm show numerous broken hairs and stumps, desquamation, and usually symptoms of mild inflammatory action. In doubtful cases recourse should be had to the microscope.

What is the prognosis in alopecia areata?

The disease is often rebellious, but in children and young adults the prognosis is almost invariably favorable, permanent loss of hair being uncommon. The same holds true, but to a much less extent, with the disease as occurring in those of more advanced age. In extensive cases—those in which the hair of the entire scalp finally [Pg 186] entirely disappears, and sometimes involves all hairy parts—the prognosis is unfavorable. Only exceptionally does recovery ensue in such instances.

The uncertain duration, however, must be borne in mind; months, and in some instances several years, may elapse before complete restoration of hair takes place. Relapses are not uncommon.

How is alopecia areata treated?

By both constitutional and local measures, the former having in view the invigoration of the nervous system, and the latter a stimulating and parasiticidal action of the affected areas.

Give the constitutional treatment.

Arsenic is perhaps the most valuable remedy, while quinine, nux vomica, pilocarpine, cod-liver oil and ferruginous tonics may, in suitable cases, often be administered with benefit.

Name several remedies or combinations employed in the external treatment of alopecia areata.

Ointments of tar and sulphur of varying strength; the various mercurial ointments; the tar oils, either pure or with alcohol; stimulating lotions, containing varying proportions, singly or in combination, of tincture of capsicum, tincture of cantharides, aqua ammoniæ, and oil of turpentine. The following is a safe formula, especially in dispensary and ignorant class practice:

> ℞ β-naphthol, ... ʒss-ʒj Ol. cadini, ... ʒj Ungt. sulphuris, ... q.s. ad. ...... ℥j M.

The cautious use of a five to twenty per cent. chrysarobin ointment is of value. Painting the patches with pure carbolic acid or trikresol every ten days or two weeks sometimes acts well; it should not be applied over large areas nor used in young children. Galvanization or faradization of the affected parts may also be employed, and with, occasionally, beneficial effect. Stimulation with the high-frequency current by means of the vacuum electrode is also of value. When practicable, the Finsen light can be applied with hope of benefit and cure. [Pg 187]

Atrophia Pilorum Propria.

(*Synonym:* Atrophy of the Hair.)

What do you understand by atrophy of the hair?

An atrophic, brittle, dry condition of the hair, and which may be either symptomatic or idiopathic.

Describe the several conditions met with.

As a symptomatic affection, the dry, brittle condition of the hair met with in seborrhœa, in severe constitutional diseases, and in the various vegetable parasitic affections, may be referred to.

As an idiopathic disease it is rare, consisting simply of a brittleness and an uneven and irregular formation of the hair-shaft, with a tendency to split up into filaments (*fragilitas crinium*); or there may be localized swelling and bursting of the hair-shaft, the nodes thus produced having a shining, semi-transparent appearance (*trichorrhexis nodosa*). This latter usually occurs upon the beard and moustache.

State the causes of atrophy of the hair.

The causes of the symptomatic variety are usually evident; the etiology of idiopathic atrophy is obscure, but by many is thought due to parasitism.

Fig. 39.

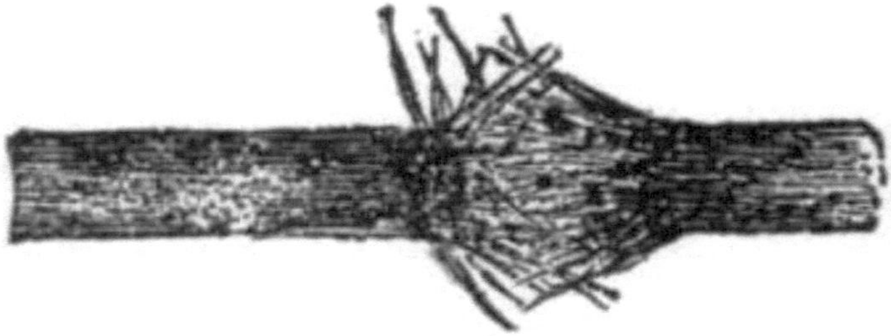

Trichorrhexis Nodosa. (*After Michelson.*)

What would be your prognosis and treatment in atrophy of the hair?

Symptomatic atrophy usually responds to proper measures, but always slowly; treatment is based upon the etiological factors.

For the idiopathic disease little, as a rule, can be done; repeated shaving or cutting the hair has, in exceptional instances, been followed by favorable results. [Pg 188]

Atrophia Unguis.

(*Synonyms:* Atrophy of the Nails; Onychatrophia.)

Describe atrophy of the nails.

The nails are soft, thin and brittle, splitting easily, and are often opaque and lustreless, and may have a worm-eaten appearance. Several or more are usually affected.

State the causes of atrophy of the nails.

The condition may be congenital or acquired, usually the latter. It may result from trauma, or be produced by certain cutaneous diseases, notably eczema and psoriasis; or it may follow injuries or diseases of the nerves. Syphilis and chronic wasting constitutional diseases may also interfere with the normal growth of the nail-substance, producing varying degrees of atrophy. The fungi of tinea trichophytina and tinea favosa at times invade these structures and lead to more or less complete disintegration—*onychomycosis*.

Fig. 40.

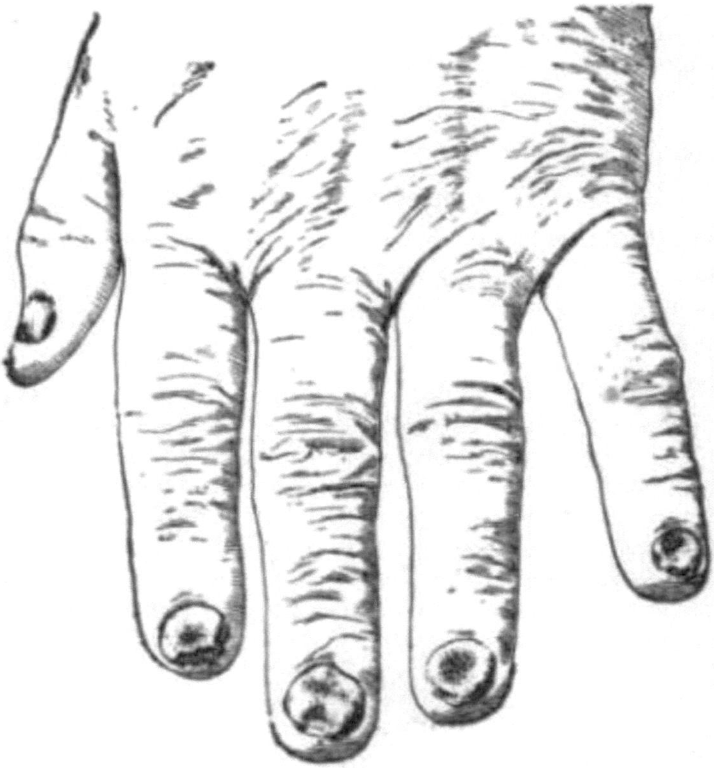

Atrophy of the Nails.

What is the treatment of atrophy of the nails?

Treatment will depend upon the cause. When it is due to eczema [Pg 189] or psoriasis, appropriate constitutional and local remedies should be prescribed. If it is the result of syphilis, mercury and potassium iodide are to be advised. In onychomycosis—an exceedingly obstinate affection—the nails should be kept closely cut and pared, and a one- to five-grain solution of corrosive sublimate applied several times a day; a lotion of sodium hyposulphite, a drachm to the ounce, is also a valuable and safe application.

Atrophia Cutis.

(*Synonyms:* Atrophoderma; Atrophy of the Skin.)

What do you understand by atrophy of the skin?

By atrophy of the skin is meant an idiopathic or symptomatic wasting or degeneration of its component elements.

State the several conditions met with.

Glossy skin, general idiopathic atrophy of the skin, parchment skin, atrophic lines and spots, senile atrophy, and the atrophy following certain cutaneous diseases.

Describe glossy skin (atrophoderma neuriticum), and state the treatment.

Glossy skin is a rare condition following an injury or disease of the nerve. It is usually seen about the fingers. The skin is hairless, faintly reddish, smooth and shining, with a varnished and thin appearance, and with a tendency to fissuring. More or less severe and persistent burning pain precedes and accompanies the atrophy.

Protective applications are called for, the disease tending slowly to spontaneous disappearance.

Describe general idiopathic atrophy of the skin, and give the treatment.

General idiopathic atrophy of the skin is extremely rare, and is characterized by a gradual, more or less general, degenerative and quantitative atrophy of the skin structures, accompanied usually with more or less discoloration and pigmentation.

Treatment is palliative and based upon indications. [Pg 190]

Describe parchment skin, and state the treatment.

Parchment skin (*xeroderma pigmentosum, angioma pigmentosum et atrophicum*) is a rare disease, the exact nature of which is not understood. It is characterized by the appearance of numerous disseminated, freckle-like pigment-spots, telangiectases, atrophied muscles, more or less shrinking and contraction of the integument, and followed, in most instances, by epitheliomatous tumors and ulceration, and finally death. It is usually slow in its course, beginning in childhood and lasting for years. It is not infrequently seen in several children of the same family.

Treatment is palliative, consisting, if necessary, of the use of protective applications and of the administration of tonics and nutrients.

Describe atrophic lines and spots.

Atrophic lines and spots (*striæ et maculæ atrophicæ*) may be idiopathic or symptomatic, the lesions consisting of scar-like or atrophic-looking, whitish lines and macules, most commonly seen on the trunk. They are smooth and glistening. Slight hyperæmia usually precedes their formation. As an idiopathic disease its course is insidious and slow, and its progress eventually stayed. The so-called *lineæ albicantes*, resulting from the stretching of the skin produced by pregnancy or tumors, and from rapid development of fat, may be mentioned as illustrating the symptomatic variety.

In course of time the atrophy becomes less conspicuous.

Describe senile atrophy.

Senile atrophy is not uncommon, the atrophy resulting, as the name inferentially implies, from advancing age. It is characterized by thinning and wasting, dryness, and a wrinkled condition, with more or less pigmentation and loss of hair. Circumscribed pigmentary deposits and seborrhœa, with degeneration, are also noted.

What several diseases of the skin are commonly followed by atrophic changes?

Favus, lupus, syphilis, leprosy, scleroderma and morphœa. [Pg 191]

CLASS VI.—NEW GROWTHS.

Keloid.

(*Synonyms:* Keloid of Alibert; Cheloid.)

Give a descriptive definition of keloid.

Keloid is a fibro-cellular new growth of the corium appearing as one or several variously-sized, irregularly-shaped, elevated, smooth, firm, pinkish or pale-reddish cicatriform lesions.

Describe the clinical appearance of keloid.

The growth begins as a small, hard, elevated, pinkish or reddish tubercle, increasing gradually, several months or years usually elapsing before the tumor reaches conspicuous size. When developed, it is one or more inches in diameter, is sharply defined, elevated, hard, rounded or oval, fungoid or crab-shaped, and firmly implanted in the skin. It is usually pinkish, pearl-white, or reddish, commonly devoid of hair, with no tendency to scaliness, and with, usually, several vessels coursing over it. In some instances it is tender, and it may be spontaneously painful.

The breast, especially over the sternal region, is a favorite site for its appearance. One, several or more may be present in the single case.

What course does keloid pursue?

Chronic; usually lasting throughout life. In rare instances spontaneous involution takes place.

State the etiology of keloid.

The causes are obscure. The growth usually takes its start from some injury or lesion of continuity; for instance, at the site of burns, cuts, acne and smallpox scars, etc.—*cicatricial keloid, false keloid*; or it may also, so it is thought, originate in normal skin—*spontaneous keloid, true keloid*.

What is the pathology of keloid?

The lesion is a connective-tissue new growth having its seat in the corium. [Pg 192]

Is there any difficulty in the diagnosis of keloid?

No. It resembles hypertrophic scar; but this latter, which is essentially keloidal, never extends beyond the line of injury.

Give the prognosis.

The growth is persistent and usually irresponsive to treatment. In some cases, however, there is eventually a tendency to spontaneous retrogression, up to a certain point at least.

What is the treatment of keloid?

Usually palliative, consisting of the continuous application of an ointment such as the following:—

> ℞ Acidi salicylici, ... gr. x-xx Emplast. plumbi, Emplast. saponis, ...āā.......... ℥iij Petrolati, ... ℥ij. M.

An ointment of ichthyol, twenty-five per cent. strength, rubbed in once or twice daily, is sometimes beneficial.

Operative measures, such as punctate and linear scarification, electrolysis and excision, are occasionally practised, but the results are rarely satisfactory and permanent; not infrequently, indeed, renewed activity in the progress of the growth is noted to follow. The *x*-ray can be tried with some hope of improvement. The administration of thyroid has been thought to have a possible influence in some instances.

Fibroma.

(*Synonyms:* Molluscum Fibrosum; Fibroma Molluscum.)

What do you understand by fibroma?

Fibroma is a connective-tissue new growth characterized by one or more sessile or pedunculated, pea- to egg-sized or larger, soft or firm, rounded, painless tumors, seated beneath and in the skin.

Describe the clinical appearances of fibroma.

The growth may be single, in which case it is apt to be pedunculated or pendulous, and attain considerable dimensions; as a result of weight or pressure surface-ulceration may occur. Or, as commonly met with, the lesions are numerous, scattered over large surface, and [Pg 193] vary in size from a pea to a cherry; the overlying skin being normal, pinkish or reddish, loose, stretched, hypertrophied or atrophied.

The tumors are painless. The general health is not involved.

Fig. 41.

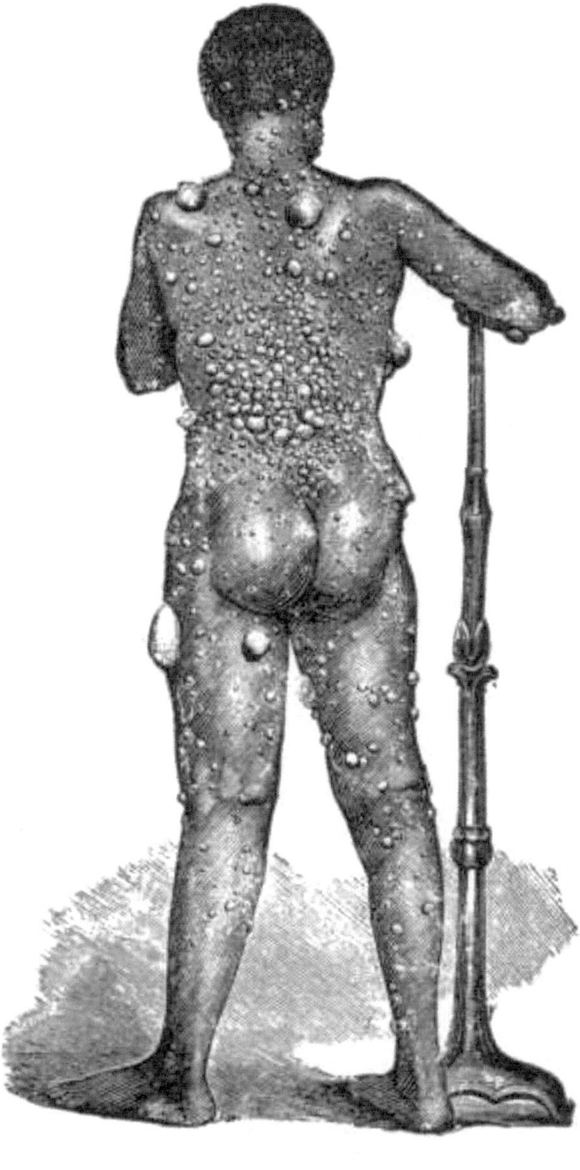

Fibroma. (*After Octerlony.*)

What is the course of fibroma?

Chronic and persistent. [Pg 194]

What is the etiology of fibroma?

The cause is not known. Heredity is often noted. The affection is not common.

State the pathology of fibroma.

The growths are variously thought to have their origin in the connective tissue of the corium, or in that of the walls of the hair-sac, or in the connective-tissue framework of the fatty tissue. Recent tumors are composed of gelatinous, newly-formed connective tissue, and the older growths of a dense, firmly-packed, fibrous tissue.

From what growths is fibroma to be differentiated?

From molluscum contagiosum, neuroma and lipoma; the first is differentiated by its central aperture or depression, neuroma by its painfulness, and lipoma by its lobulated character and soft feel.

Give the prognosis of fibroma.

The disease is persistent, and irresponsive to all treatment save operative measures.

What is the treatment of fibroma?

Treatment consists, when desired and practicable, in the removal of the growths by the knife, or in large and pedunculated tumors by the ligature or by the galvano-cautery.

Neuroma.

Describe neuroma.

Neuroma of the skin is an exceedingly rare disease, characterized by the formation of variously-sized, usually numerous, firm, immovable and elastic fibrous tubercles containing new nerve-elements, and accompanied by violent, paroxysmal pain. Their growth is slow and usually progressive. Later they are painful upon pressure. They are limited to one region.

The tumors are seated in the corium, extending into the deeper structure, and consist of nerve-fibres, yellow elastic tissue, blood vessels and lymphoid cells.

In the two cases reported, excision of the nerve-trunk gave, in one instance, permanent relief; in the other the effect was only temporary. [Pg 195]

Xanthoma.

(*Synonyms:* Vitiligoidea; Xanthelasma.)

What is xanthoma?

Xanthoma is a connective-tissue new growth characterized by the formation of yellowish, circumscribed, irregularly-shaped, variously-sized, non-indurated, flat or raised patches or tubercles.

Name the two varieties met with.

The macular or flat (*xanthoma planum*) and the tubercular (*xanthoma tuberculatum* or *tuberosum*). In some instances both varieties (*xanthoma multiplex*) are seen in the same individual.

Describe the clinical appearances of xanthoma planum.

The macular or flat variety is usually seen about the eyelids. It consists of one, several or more small or large, smooth, opaque, sharply-defined, often slightly raised, yellowish patches, looking not unlike pieces of chamois-skin implanted in the skin.

Describe the clinical appearances of xanthoma tuberosum.

The tubercular variety is commonly met with upon the neck, trunk and extremities. It occurs as small, raised, isolated, yellowish nodules, or as patches made up of aggregations of millet-seed-sized or larger tubercles. The lesions may be few or they may exist in great numbers.

What is the course of xanthoma?

Extremely slow; after reaching a certain development the growths may remain stationary.

State the etiology of xanthoma.

The causes are obscure. Jaundice not infrequently precedes and accompanies its development, especially in the tubercular variety. The disease is uncommon, and is usually seen in middle and advanced life, and more frequently in women. In some cases (*xanthoma diabeticorum*) of general xanthoma diabetes is the causative factor.

What is the pathology of xanthoma?

It is a benign, connective-tissue new growth, with concomitant or subsequent, but usually partial, fatty degeneration. [Pg 196]

Give the prognosis of xanthoma.

The condition is persistent, and usually irresponsive to all treatment save destructive or operative measures.

What is the treatment of xanthoma?

Treatment consists, in suitable cases, of excision; in some instances, electrolysis is serviceable. Applications of trichloracetic acid cautiously made are sometimes of value. In that form of general xanthoma due to diabetes the treatment of this latter condition will materially and sometimes completely remove the eruption.

Myoma.

(*Synonyms:* Myoma Cutis; Dermatomyoma; Liomyoma Cutis.)

Describe myoma.

The disease is rare, and consists usually of one or several (exceptionally numerous), variously-sized tumors of the skin, made up of smooth muscular fibres. They are flat, rounded, oval or pedunculated, and have a smooth surface and a pale-red color; as a rule, they are painless.

The growth is benign, and consists essentially of a new formation of unstriped muscular fibres; but it may also be composed largely of connective tissue (*fibromyoma*); or it may contain an abundance of bloodvessels (*myoma telangiectodes, angiomyoma*); or there may be lymphatic involvement (*lymphangiomyoma*).

Angioma.

(*Synonyms:* Nævus Vasculosus; Nævus Sanguineus.)

Give a definition of angioma.

Angioma is a congenital hypertrophy of the vascular tissues of the corium and subcutaneous tissue. Exceptionally it makes its appearance a few weeks or a month after birth.

Into what two classes may angiomata be roughly grouped?

The flat (or non-elevated) and the prominent (or elevated).

Describe the flat, or non-elevated, variety of angioma.

The flat, or non-elevated, angioma (*nævus flammeus, nævus simplex, angioma simplex, capillary nævus*) may be pin-head- to bean-sized; or it may involve an area of several inches in diameter, and, [Pg 197] exceptionally, a whole region. It is of a bright- or dark-red color, and is met with most frequently about the face. In some instances it extends after birth, reaches a certain size and then remains stationary; occasionally, when involving a small area, it undergoes involution and disappears.

The so-called *port-wine mark* is included in this group.

Describe the prominent, or elevated, variety of angioma.

The prominent variety (*venous nœvus, angioma cavernosum, nœvus tuberosus*) is variously-sized, often considerably elevated, clearly-defined, compressible, smooth or lobulated, and of a dark, purple color; it may, also, be erectile and pulsating. The growth is usually a single formation, and is met with upon all parts of the body.

What is the pathology of angioma?

It is a new growth, consisting of a variable hypertrophy of the cutaneous and subcutaneous arterial and venous bloodvessels, with or without an increase of the connective tissue.

Give the treatment of angioma.

In some instances, especially in infants, painting the parts repeatedly with collodion or liquor plumbi subacetatis will act favorably. For well-established, small, capillary nævi electrolysis or puncturing with a red-hot needle or with a needle charged with nitric acid may be employed; for "port-wine mark" frequent and closely contiguous electrolytic punctures are occasionally followed by a slight diminution in color. For the *prominent growths*, vaccination, the ligature, puncturing with the galvano-cautery, and excision are variously resorted to.

In recent years applications of liquid air and carbon dioxide have proved of service in some cases.

Telangiectasis.

Describe telangiectasis.

Telangiectasis consists of a new growth or enlargement of the cutaneous capillaries, usually appearing during middle adult life, and seated, for the most part, about the face.

To what extent may telangiectasis develop?

It may be limited to a red dot or point, with several small radiating [Pg 198] capillaries (*nævus araneus, spider nævus*), or a whole region, usually the face, may show numerous scattered or closely-set capillary enlargements or new formations (*rosacea*). The latter is frequently associated with acne (*acne rosacea*).

The etiology is obscure.

What is the treatment of telangiectasis?

Destruction of the vessels by electrolysis or by the knife. (See treatment of acne rosacea.)

Lymphangioma.

(*Synonym:* Lymphangiectodes.)

Describe lymphangioma.

Lymphangioma is a rare disease, consisting of localized dilatations of the lymphatic vessels, appearing as discrete or aggregated pin-head or pea-sized, compressible, hollow, tubercle-like elevations, of a pinkish or faint lilac color, and occurring for the most part about the trunk. It is of slow but usually progressive development, and is unaccompanied by subjective symptoms.

A rare condition, Kaposi described as lymphangioma tuberosum multiplex, characterized by more or less solid, somewhat cystic, pearly to pinkish red, sometimes crowded lesions, is now known to be "benign cystic epithelioma"; its most common site is the face. While called "benign," ulcerative action may eventually ensue.

Treatment, when demanded, consists of operative measures.

Rhinoscleroma.

Describe rhinoscleroma.

Rhinoscleroma is a rare and obscure disease, slow but progressive in its course, characterized by the development of an irregular, dense and hard, flattened, tubercular, non-ulcerating, cellular new growth, having its seat about the nose and contiguous parts. The overlying skin is normal in color, or it may be light- or dark-brown or reddish. Marked disfigurement and closure, partial or complete, of the nasal [Pg 199] orifices gradually results. It is met with chiefly in Austria and Germany.

Treatment, consisting of partial or complete extirpation, is rarely permanent in its results, the disease tending to recur.

Lupus Erythematosus.

(*Synonyms:* Lupus Erythematodes; Lupus Sebaceus; Seborrhœa Congestiva.)

What is lupus erythematosus?

Lupus erythematosus may be roughly defined as a mildly to moderately inflammatory superficial new-growth formation, characterized by one, several, or more circumscribed, variously sized and shaped, pinkish or dark red patches, covered slightly, and more or less irregularly, with adherent grayish or yellowish scales.

Upon what parts is lupus erythematosus observed?

Its common site is the face, usually the nose and cheeks, with a tendency toward symmetry; it is often limited to these parts, but may occasionally be seen upon other regions, more especially the lips, ears, and scalp. In rare instances a great part of the general surface may become involved.

Describe the symptoms of lupus erythematosus.

Usually the disease begins as one or several rounded, circumscribed, pin-head- to pea-sized lesions; slightly scaly, somewhat elevated, and of a pinkish, reddish or violaceous color. They slowly, or somewhat rapidly, increase in area, and after attaining variable size remain stationary; or they may progress and coalesce, and in this manner sooner or later involve considerable surface. The patches are sharply defined against the sound skin by an elevated border, while the central portion is somewhat depressed and usually atrophic. More or less thickening and infiltration are observed. *There is no tendency to ulceration*. The scaliness is, as a rule, scanty. The gland-ducts are enlarged, patulous or plugged with sebaceous and epithelial matter.

The subjective symptoms of burning and itching are usually slight and often wanting.

What course does lupus erythematosus pursue?

As a rule, the disease is persistent, although somewhat variable. [Pg 200] At times the patches retrogress, involution taking place with or without slight sieve-like atrophy or scarring.

State the causes of lupus erythematosus.

The etiology is obscure. Some observers believe it to be a variety of cutaneous tuberculosis. It is essentially a disease of adult and middle age; is more common in women, and more frequent in those having a tendency to disorders of the sebaceous glands. It may, in fact, begin as a seborrhœa.

What is the pathology?

It was formerly considered a new growth, but recent opinion tends toward regarding it as a chronic inflammation of the cutis, superinducing degenerative and atrophic changes. Variable œdema of the prickle layer and of the cutis is found. There is no tendency to pus formation.

Fig. 42.

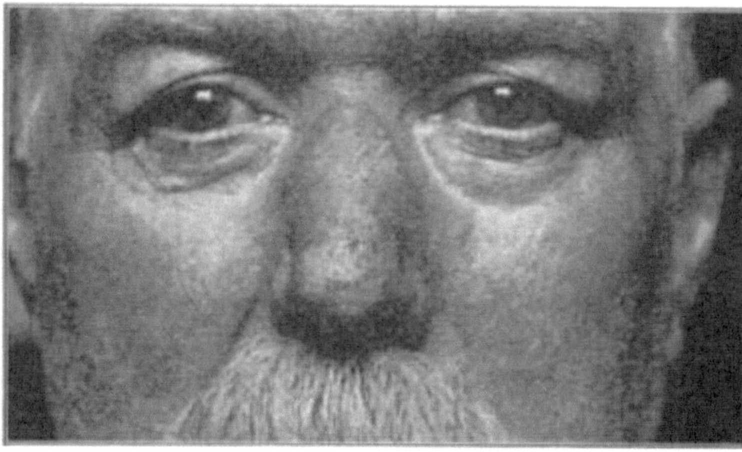

Lupus Erythematosus.

Is there any difficulty in the diagnosis of lupus erythematosus?

As a rule, not, as the features of the disease—the sharply circumscribed outline, the reddish or violaceous color, the elevated border, the tendency to central depression and atrophy, the plugged up or patulous sebaceous ducts, the adherent grayish or yellowish scales, [Pg 201] together with the region attacked (usually the nose and cheeks)— are characteristic.

State the prognosis of lupus erythematosus.

The disease is often capricious and extremely rebellious to treatment; some cases, up to a certain point at least, yield readily, and occasionally a tendency to spontaneous disappearance is observed; a complete cure is, however, it must be confessed, rather rare. The disease in nowise compromises the general health. In those rare instances of generalized disease the patient has usually died from an intercurrent tuberculosis.

How is lupus erythematosus to be treated?

The general health is to be looked after and systemic treatment prescribed, if indicated. As a rule, constitutional remedies exert little, if any, influence, but exceptionally, cod-liver oil, arsenic, phosphorus, salicin, quinine, or potassium iodide proves of service.

Locally, according to the case, soothing remedies, stimulating applications and destruction of the growth by caustics or operative measures are to be employed. (*Try the milder applications first.*)

Mention the stimulating applications commonly employed.

Washing the parts energetically with tincture of sapo viridis, rinsing and applying a soothing ointment, such as cold cream or vaseline.

A lotion containing zinc sulphate and potassium sulphuret thoroughly dabbed on the parts morning and evening:—

> ℞ Zinci sulphatis, Potassii sulphurati, ...āā........... ʒi-ʒiv Glycerinæ, ... ♏iv Aquæ, ... f℥iv. M.

The calamine-and-zinc oxide lotion used in acute eczema is also often extremely valuable.

Lotions of ichthyol and of resorcin, five to sixty grains to the ounce; ichthyol in ointment, five- to twenty-per-cent. strength, is also useful.

Painting the patches with pure carbolic acid; repeating a day or two after the crusts have fallen off.

The continuous application of mercurial plaster. [Pg 202] Sulphur and tar ointments, officinal strength or weakened with lard, and also the following:—

> ℞ Ol. cadini, Alcoholis, Saponis viridis, ...āā............. ʒiiss. M.

(This is to be rubbed in, in small quantity, once or twice daily, and later a soothing remedy applied.)

In recent years both the *x*-ray and Finsen light have been used with variable success. Repeated applications of the high-frequency current, with the vacuum electrode, have also proved serviceable.

Cautious applications of liquid air or carbon dioxide have also been used with some success in the past few years.

When are destructive and operative measures justifiable?

In obstinate, sluggish, and long-persistent patches, and then only after other methods of treatment have failed. (Remember that a patch or patches of the disease *may* disappear in course of time spontaneously, and occasionally *without leaving a scar*.)

State the methods of treatment commonly used in obstinate, sluggish and persistent patches of lupus erythematosus.

Cauterization—with nitrate of silver, with applications of pyrogallic acid in ointment or in liquor gutta-perchæ, fifteen to thirty per cent. strength, and with solutions (cautiously employed) of caustic potash, and exceptionally with the galvano-cautery.

Fig. 43.

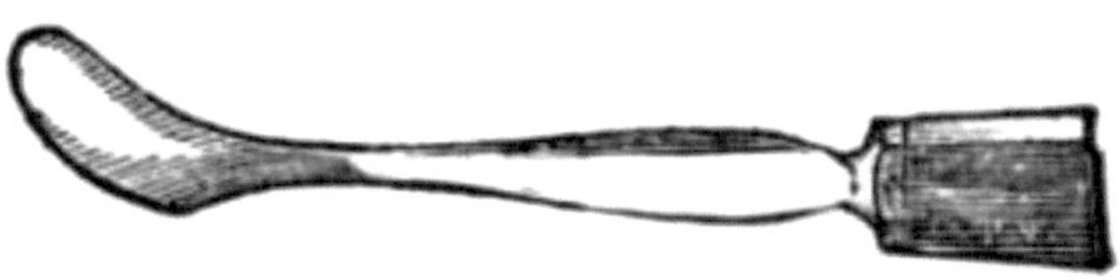

Single Scarifier.

Fig. 44.

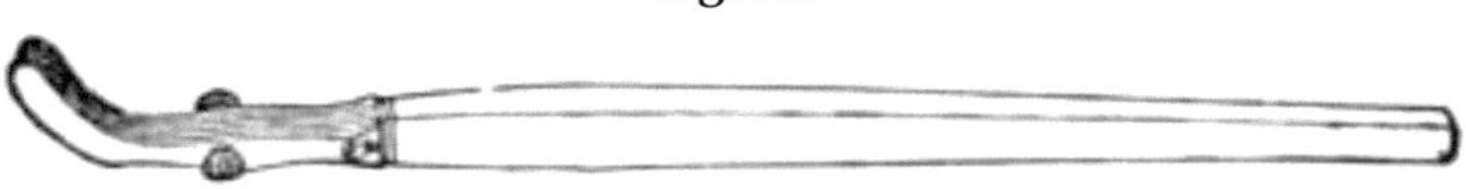

Multiple Scarifier. (*As modified by Van Harlingen.*)

[Pg 203] Operative—scarification, either punctate or linear, and erosion with the curette. (See treatment of lupus vulgaris.)

Lupus Vulgaris.

(*Synonyms:* Lupus; Lupus Exedens; Lupus Vorax; Tuberculosis of the Skin.)

What do you understand by lupus vulgaris?

Lupus vulgaris is a cellular new growth, characterized by variously-sized, soft, reddish-brown, papular, tubercular and infiltrated patches, usually terminating in ulceration and scarring.

Upon what region is lupus vulgaris usually observed?

The face, especially the nose, but any part may be invaded. The area involved may be small or quite extensive, usually the former.

At what age is the disease noted?

In many cases it begins in childhood or early adult life, but as it is persistent and tends to relapse, it may be met with at any age.

Describe the earlier symptoms of lupus vulgaris.

The disease begins by the development of several or more pinhead to small pea-sized, deep-seated, brownish-red or yellowish tubercles, having their seat in the deeper part of the corium, and which are somewhat softer and looser in texture than normal tissue. As the disease progresses, variously-sized and shaped aggregations or patches result, covered with thin and imperfectly-formed epidermis.

What changes do the lupus tubercles or infiltrations undergo?

The lesions, having attained a certain size or development, may remain so for a time, but sooner or later retrogressive changes occur: the matured papules or tubercles, or infiltrated patches, slowly disappear by absorption, fatty degeneration, and exfoliation, leaving a yellowish or brownish pigmentation, usually with more or less atrophy or cicatricial-tissue formation—*lupus exfoliativus*; or disintegration and destruction result, terminating in ulceration—*lupus exedens, lupus exulcerans*. This latter is the more usual course.

Describe the clinical appearances and behavior of the lupus ulcerations.

They are rounded, shallow excavations, with soft and reddish borders. In exceptional instances exuberant granulations appear—

[Pg 204] *lupus hypertrophicus*; or papillary outgrowths are noted—*lupus verrucosus*. The ulcerations secrete a variable amount of pus, usually slight in quantity, which leads to more or less crust formation; later, however, cicatricial tissue, generally of a *firm and fibrous* character, results.

Fig. 45.

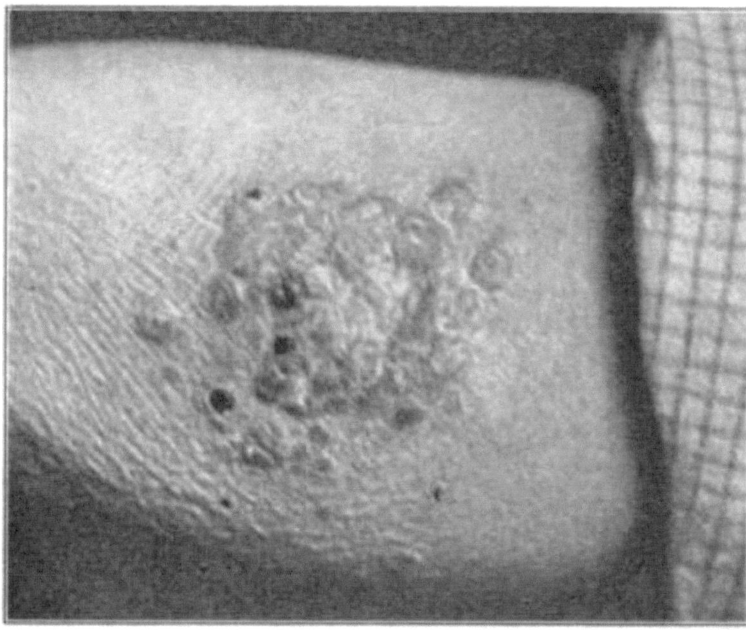

Lupus of Arm.

In what manner does the disease spread?

The patches spread by the appearance of new tubercles, or infiltrations at the peripheral portion. New islets and areas of disease may continue to make their appearance from time to time, usually upon contiguous parts.

Are the mucous membranes of the mouth, throat and larynx ever involved?

In some instances, and either primarily or secondarily.

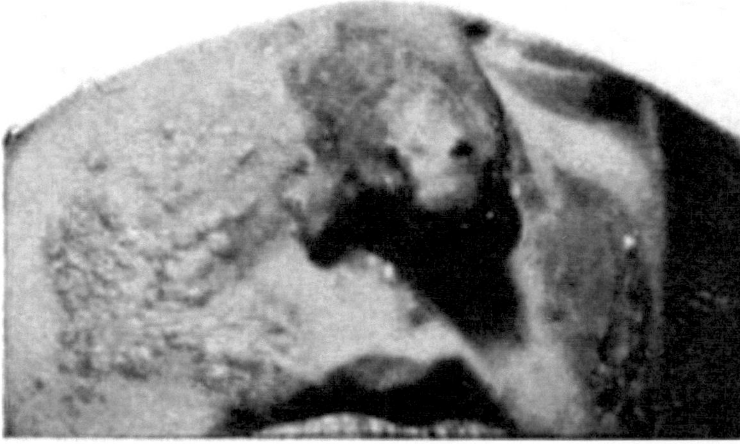

Lupus Vulgaris.

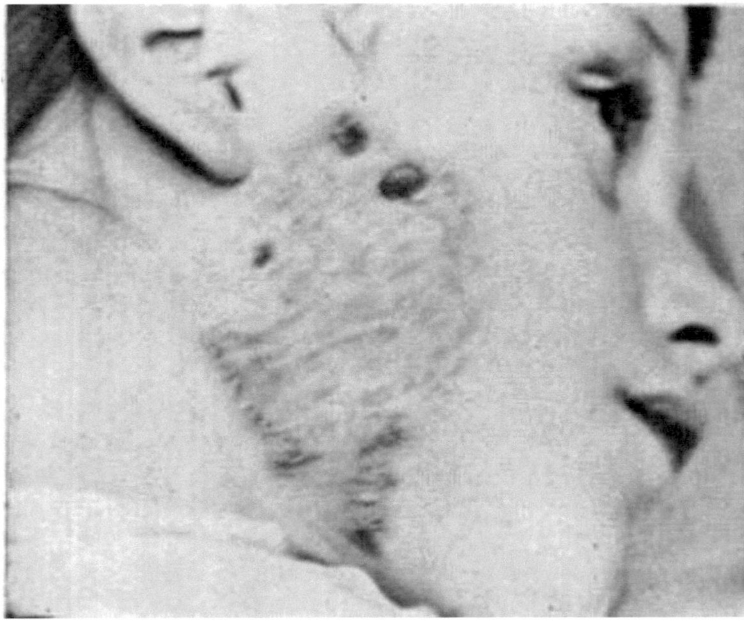

Lupus Vulgaris.

[Pg 205]

Is the bone tissue ever involved in lupus vulgaris?

No.

What course does lupus vulgaris pursue?

It is slowly but, as a rule, steadily progressive. Several years or more may elapse before the area of disease is conspicuous.

What is the cause of lupus vulgaris?

It is now known to be due to the invasion of the cutaneous structures by the tubercle bacillus; in short, a tuberculosis of the skin. It is not infrequently observed in the strumous and debilitated. It is entirely independent of syphilis.

What is the pathology of lupus vulgaris?

According to recent investigations, the infiltrations of lupus are due chiefly to cell-proliferation and outgrowth from the protoplasmic walls and adventitia of the bloodvessels and lymphatics. The fibrous-tissue network, vessels and a portion of the cell infiltration are thus produced, the fixed and wandering connective-tissue cells of the inflamed stroma of the cutis being responsible for the other portion of the new growth (Robinson).

State the diagnostic features of lupus vulgaris.

In a typical, developed patch of lupus are to be seen:—cicatricial formation, usually of a fibrous and tough character; ulcerations; the yellowish-brown tubercles and infiltration; and the characteristic soft, small, yellowish or reddish-brown, cutaneous and subcutaneous points and tubercles.

How does the tubercular syphiloderm differ from lupus vulgaris?

The tubercular syphiloderm is much more rapid in its course, the ulceration is deeper and the discharge copious and often offensive; the scarring is soft, and, compared to the amount of ulceration, but slightly disfiguring; and it is, for obvious reasons, a disease of adult or late life. The history, together with other evidences of previous or concomitant symptoms of syphilis, will often aid in the differentiation.

How does epithelioma differ from lupus vulgaris?

The edges of the epitheliomatous ulcer are hard, elevated and waxy; the base is uneven, the secretion thin, scanty and apt to be [Pg 206] streaked with blood; the ulceration usually starts from one point, and is often painful; the tissue destruction may be considerable; there is little, if any, tendency to the formation of cicatricial tissue; and, finally, it is usually a disease of advanced age.

In what respects does lupus erythematosus differ from lupus vulgaris?

Lupus erythematosus has no papules, tubercles or ulceration.

How does acne rosacea differ from lupus vulgaris?

Acne rosacea is characterized by hyperæmia, dilated vessels, papules, pustules, the absence of ulceration, and a different history.

State the prognosis of lupus vulgaris.

Lupus vulgaris is always a chronic disease, often exceedingly rebellious to treatment, and one that calls for a guarded opinion. Relapses are not uncommon.

Fig. 46.

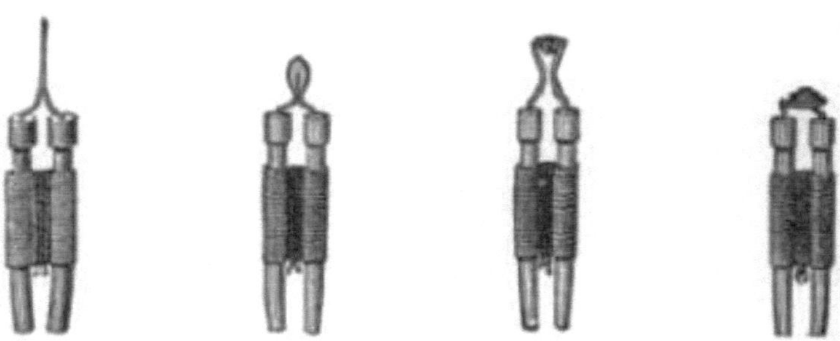

Galvano-cautery Needle, Knife and Spiral Points. (*As devised by Bésnier.*)

The general health usually remains good, but in some instances death by tuberculosis of the lungs has been noted.

Is external or internal treatment called for in lupus vulgaris?

Always external, and not infrequently constitutional also.

What is the constitutional treatment?

The general health must be cared for; good, nutritious food, fresh air and out-door exercise, together with, in many cases, the administration of such remedies as cod-liver oil, potassium iodide, iron and quinine, are of therapeutic importance. Tuberculin may be tried in severe and obstinate cases, but its use is not without danger. [Pg 207]

State the object of local treatment.

The destruction or removal of the diseased tissue.

May milder methods of treatment sometimes prove beneficial and even curative?

Exceptionally, mercurial plaster, corrosive-sublimate lotion and ointment (gr. j to ℥ j), a plaster containing five to fifteen per cent. of salicylic acid and creasote, repeated paintings with carbolic acid, and the constant application of lead plaster containing twenty per cent. of ichthyol, are valuable.

Fig. 47.

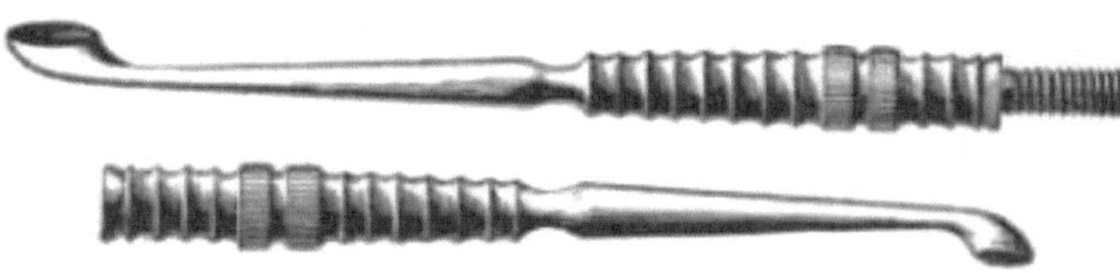

Double Curette.

Of the milder methods, those most in vogue to-day are the *Finsen light* and *x-ray*. Either proves extremely valuable in some cases, but the Finsen method is the favorite method.

What methods are commonly employed for the rapid removal or destruction of lupus tissue?

Cauterization, scarification, erasion and excision are variously practised; the particular method depending, in great measure, upon the extent of the disease, the part involved, and other circumstances.

Name the several caustics, and state how they are employed.

Pyrogallic acid, used as an ointment:—

> ℞ Ac. pyrogallici, ... ʒij Emplast. plumbi, ... ʒj Cerat. resinsæ, ... ʒv. M.

It is applied for one or two weeks. Every several days the parts are poulticed, the slough thus removed, and the ointment reapplied, and so on until the diseased tissue has been destroyed. It is useful in those cases in which a mild and comparatively painless caustic is advisable. In most cases several repetitions of this plan are necessary. [Pg 208] *Arsenious acid,* employed as an ointment—

> ℞ Ac. arseniosi, ... gr. xx Hydrarg. sulphid. rub., ... gr. lx Ungt. aquæ rosæ, ... ℥i. M.

It is painful but thorough; it is spread on lint and renewed daily. The action is usually sufficient in three days, and the parts are then poulticed until the slough comes away, after which a simple dressing is employed. Its application is advisable for a small area only—not more than four square inches—as absorption is possible.

Galvano-cautery.—The diseased tissue is destroyed by numerous punctures with a red-heated point or by linear incision with a red-heated knife. It is often a practicable and satisfactory method. The Paquelin cautery and liquid air and carbon dioxide also have their advocates.

Describe the operative measures employed in the removal of lupus tissue.

Linear Scarification.—The parts are thoroughly cross-tracked, cutting through the diseased tissue, and subsequently a simple salicylated ointment applied. The operation is repeated from time to time, and as a result the new growth undergoes retrogressive changes, and cicatrization takes place.

Punctate Scarification.—By means of a simple or multiple-pointed instrument numerous closely-set punctures are made, and repeated from time to time, usually with the same action and result as from linear scarification.

Erasion.—The parts are thoroughly scraped with a curette, and a supplementary caustic application made, either with caustic potash or several days' use of the pyrogallic-acid ointment. The result is usually satisfactory.

The dental-burr is also useful in breaking up discrete tubercles.

Excision.—This is an effective method if the disease consists of a small pea- or bean-sized circumscribed patch.

Of these various operative methods those now most favored are erasion and excision, punctate and linear scarification methods are now rarely employed. [Pg 209]

Tuberculosis Cutis. [D]

(*Synonym:* Scrofuloderma.)

[D] The most important clinical variety of this class is lupus vulgaris, which is considered above, separately, at some length.

What do you understand by tuberculosis cutis?

The term is applied to those peculiar suppurative and ulcerative conditions of the skin due to the tubercle bacilli.

How does the common type of tuberculosis cutis begin?

The most common type of tuberculous ulceration or involvement of the skin usually results by extension from an underlying caseating and suppurating lymphatic gland; or it may have its origin as subcutaneous tubercles independently of these structures. It tends to spread, and may involve an area of one or several inches.

Fig. 48.

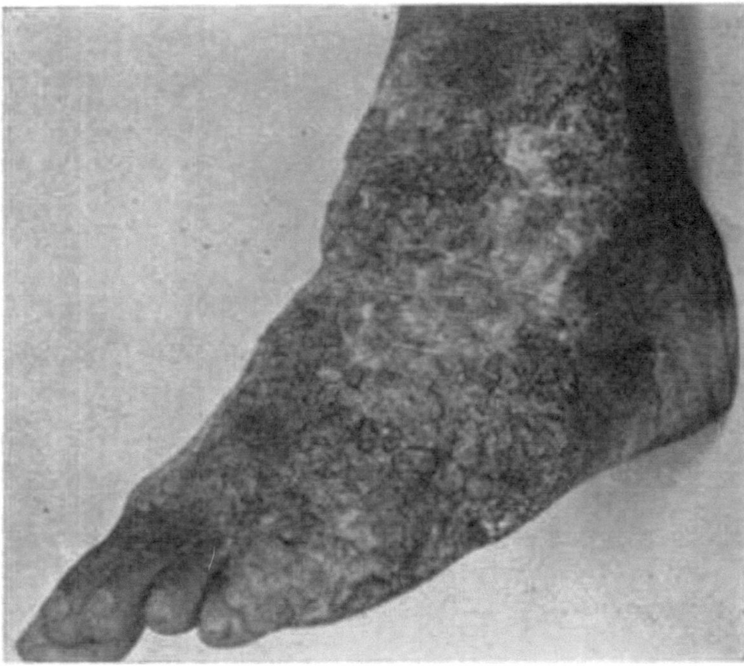

Tuberculosis Verrucosa Cutis (Negro).

[Pg 210]

What are the clinical appearances and behavior of this type of tuberculous ulceration?

It is usually superficial, has thin, red, undermined edges of a violaceous color, and an irregular base with granulations covered scantily with pus. As a rule, it spreads gradually as a simple ulceration, with but slight, if any, outlying infiltration. Subjective symptoms of a painful or troublesome character are rarely present. Its course is usually progressive but slow and chronic.

Other symptoms of tuberculosis are commonly to be found.

Are other forms of tuberculosis cutis met with?

A papulo-pustular eruption is sometimes observed, especially on the upper extremities and face; sluggish and chronic in character and leaving small pit-like scars; has been known as the *small pustular scrofuloderma.*

Fig. 49.

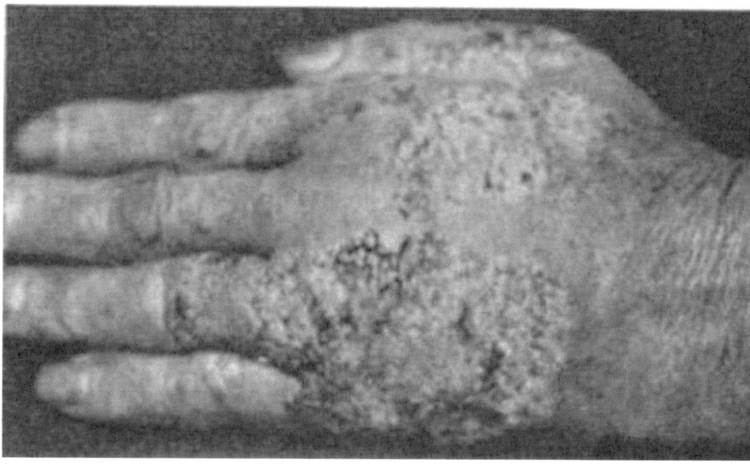

Tuberculosis Verrucosa Cutis (patient had a coexistent pulmonary tuberculosis).

An ulcerative papillomatous or verrucous tuberculosis of the skin (tuberculosis verrucosa cutis) is also occasionally noted, most commonly seated upon the lower leg or the back of the hand. It may be slight or extensive. Its mildest phase is the so-called verruca necrogenica. [Pg 211]

Describe verruca necrogenica.

Verruca necrogenica is a rare, localized, papillary or wart-like formation, occurring usually about the knuckles or other parts of the hand.

It begins, as a rule, as a small, papule-like growth, increasing gradually in area, and when well advanced appears as a pea, dime-sized or larger, somewhat inflammatory, elevated, flat, warty mass, with usually a tendency to slight pus-formation between the hypertrophied papillæ; the surface may be horny or it may be crusted. It tends to enlarge slowly and is usually persistent, but it at times undergoes involution.

Fig. 50.

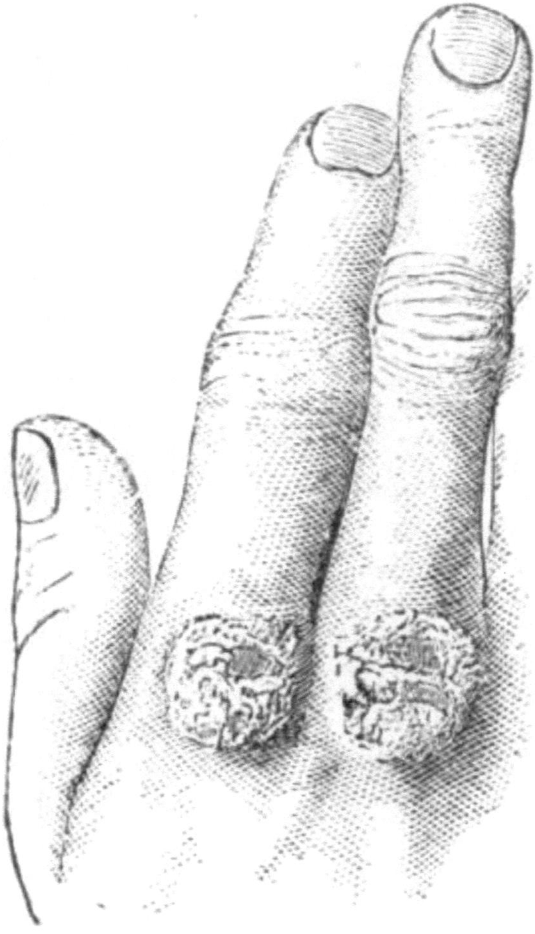

Tuberculosis Cutis (Verruca Necrogenica). (*After Model in Guy's Museum.*)

State the etiology.

Heredity, insufficient and unwholesome food, impure air, and the like are predisposing. The tubercle bacillus is the immediate exciting cause.

The disease usually appears in childhood or early adult life, and not infrequently follows in the wake of some severe systemic disease. Etiologically it is identical in nature with lupus.

How is the tuberculous ulcer to be differentiated from syphilis?

By the peculiar character of the tuberculous ulceration, the absence of outlying tubercles and infiltration, together with its history, course, and often the presence of other tuberculous symptoms. [Pg 212]

State the prognosis.

These various types of tuberculosis cutis are, as a rule, more amenable to treatment than that form known as lupus vulgaris (*q. v.*).

What is the treatment of these forms of tuberculosis cutis?

Constitutional remedies, such as cod-liver oil, iodide of iron or other ferruginous tonics, together with good food and pure air; phosphorus one-hundredth to one-fiftieth of a grain three times daily is also of benefit in some cases.

The local treatment consists in thorough curetting and the subsequent application of a mildly stimulating ointment. The several other plans of external treatment employed in lupus (*q. v.*) are also variously practised. In recent years the *x*-ray and Finsen light plans have, in a measure, supplanted the previous methods of treatment. They are slow, however, and might be, especially the *x*-ray, more satisfactorily employed as a supplementary measure.

Ainhum.

Describe ainhum.

Ainhum is a disease of the African race, met with chiefly in Brazil, the West Indies, and Africa, and consists of a slow but gradual linear strangulation of one or more of the toes, especially the smallest, resulting, eventually, in spontaneous amputation. The affected toes themselves undergo fatty degeneration, often with increase in size, and are, when strangulation is well advanced, considerably misshapen. The nature of the disease is obscure.

Treatment consists, in the early stages, of incision through the constricting band; when the disease is well advanced, amputation is the sole recourse.

Mycetoma.

(*Synonyms:* Fungous Foot of India; Madura Foot; Podelcoma.)

Describe mycetoma.

It is a disease involving usually the foot, and is met with chiefly in India. It is characterized by swelling and the formation of tubercular or nodular lesions which break down and form the external openings of sinuses which lead to the interior of the affected part. These discharge, and are studded with, whitish granules or black, roe-like masses, mixed with a sanious or sero-purulent fluid. The [Pg 213] whole part is gradually disintegrated, the process lasting indefinitely. Its nature is obscure; it is thought to be due to a fungus.

Treatment consists in the early stages, when the disease is limited, of thorough curetting and cauterization; later, after the part is more or less involved, amputation, at a point well up beyond the disease, becomes necessary. Potassium iodide internally may exert a favorable influence.

Perforating Ulcer of the Foot.

Describe perforating ulcer of the foot.

Perforating ulcer of the foot is a rare disease, consisting of an indolent and usually painless sinus leading down to diseased bone. The external opening, which is through the centre of a corn-like formation, is small, and may or may not show the presence of granulations. The affected part is commonly more or less anæsthetic and of subnormal temperature. One or several may be present, either on one or both feet. The most common site is over the articulation of the metatarsal bone with the phalanx of the first or last toe. The disease is dependent upon impairment or degeneration of the central, truncal or peripheral nerves.

What is to be said in regard to the prognosis and treatment?

Treatment, which is, as a rule, unsatisfactory, consists in the maintenance of absolute rest, and the use of antiseptic and stimulating applications. Amputation is also resorted to, but even this is at times futile, as a new sinus may appear upon the stump.

Syphilis Cutanea.

(*Synonyms:* Syphiloderma; Dermatosyphilis; Syphilis of the Skin.)

In what various types may syphilis manifest itself upon the integument?

Syphilis may show itself as a macular, papular (rarely vesicular), pustular, bullous, tubercular and gummatous eruption; or the eruption may be, in a measure, of a mixed type. [Pg 214]

In what respects do the early (or secondary) eruptions of syphilis differ from those following several years or more after the contraction of the disease?

The early or secondary eruptions are more or less generalized, with rarely any attempt at special configuration. Their appearance is often preceded by symptoms of systemic disturbance, such as fever, loss of appetite, muscular pains and headache; and accompanied by concomitant signs of the disease, such as enlargement of the lymphatic glands, sore throat, mucous patches, falling of the hair and rheumatic pains.

State the distinguishing characters of the late eruptions.

The late eruptions (those following one or more years after the contraction of the disease) are usually of tubercular, gummatous or ulcerative type; are limited in extent, and have a marked tendency to appear in circular, semicircular or crescentic forms or groups. Pain in the bones, bone lesions and other symptoms may or may not be present.

What is the color of syphilitic lesions?

Usually, a dull brownish-red or ham-red, with at times a yellowish cast.

Are there any subjective symptoms in syphilitic eruptions?

As a rule, no; but in exceptional instances of the generalized eruptions, more especially in negroes, there may be slight itching.

Describe the macular, or erythematous, eruption of syphilis.

The *macular syphiloderm* is a general eruption, showing itself usually six or eight weeks after the appearance of the chancre. It consists of small or large, commonly pea- or bean-sized, rounded or irregularly-shaped, not infrequently slightly raised, macules. When well established they do not entirely disappear under pressure. At first a pale-pink or dull, violaceous red, they later become yellowish or coppery. The eruption is generally profuse; the face, backs of the hands and feet may escape. It persists several weeks or one or two months; as a rule, it is rapidly responsive to treatment.

How would you distinguish the macular syphiloderm from measles, rötheln and tinea versicolor?

Measles is to be differentiated by its catarrhal symptoms, fever, form and situation of the eruption; rötheln, by its small, roundish, [Pg 215] confluent pinkish or reddish patches, its precursory pyrexic symptoms, its epidemic nature, and short duration; tinea versicolor by its scaliness, peripheral growth, distribution and history.

And, finally, by the absence or presence of other symptoms of syphilis.

Fig. 51.

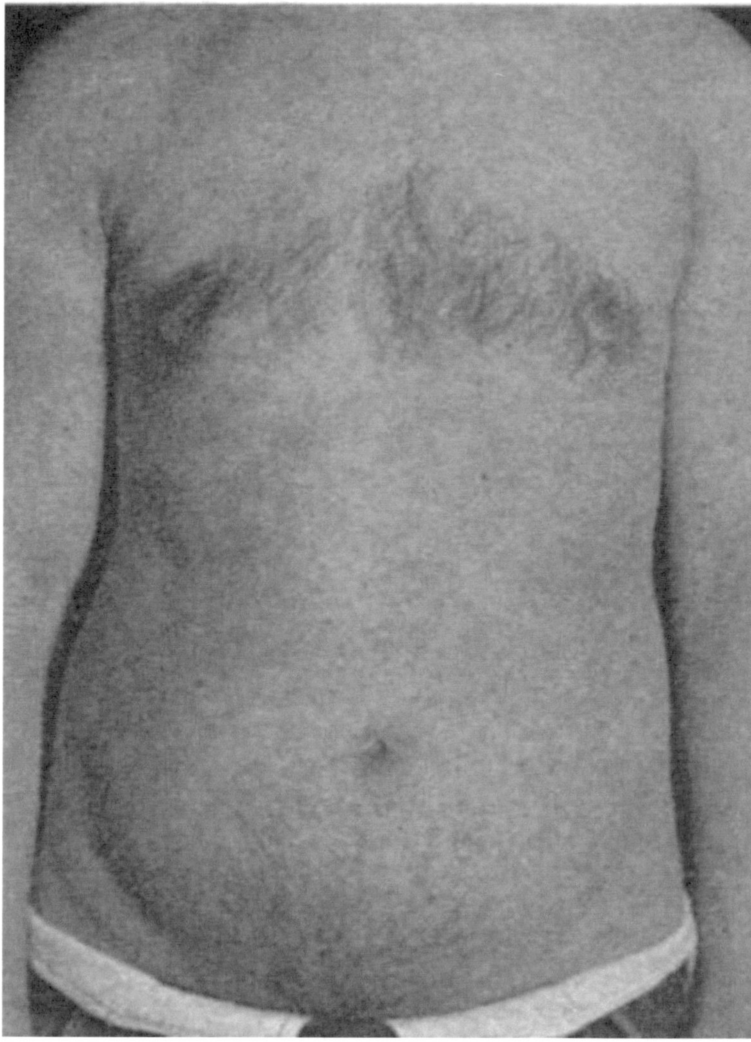

Macular Syphiloderm.

What several varieties of the papular eruption of syphilis are met with?

There are two forms of the papular eruption—the small and large; those of the latter type may undergo various modifications.

Describe the small-papular eruption of syphilis.

The *small-papular syphiloderm* (*miliary papular syphiloderm*) usually shows itself in the third or fourth month of the disease, and [Pg 216] consists of a more or less generalized eruption of disseminated or grouped, firm, rounded or acuminated pin-head to millet-seed-sized papules, with smooth or slightly scaly summits, and in some lesions showing pointed pustulation. Scattered minute pustules and some large papules are usually present. The eruption is profuse, most abundant upon the trunk and limbs; and in the early part of the outbreak is of a bright- or dull-red color, later assuming a violaceous or brownish tint. It runs a chronic course, is somewhat rebellious to treatment, and displays a tendency to relapse.

Fig. 52.

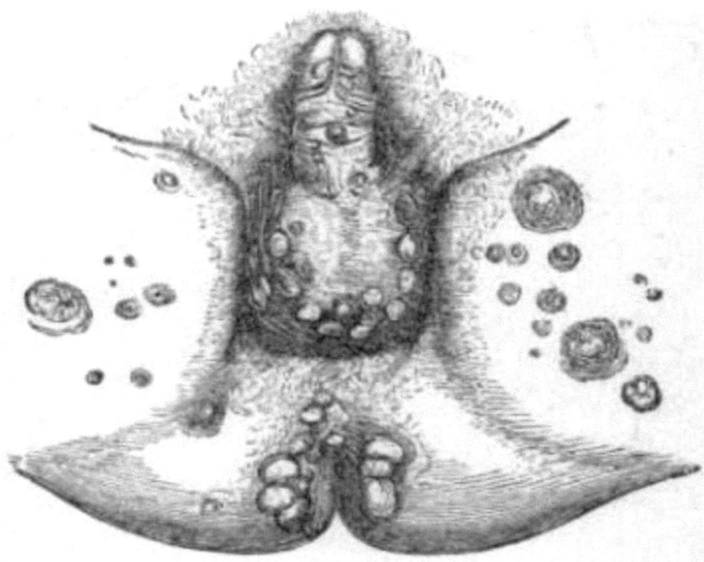

Moist Papules. (*After Miller.*)

How would you distinguish the small-papular syphiloderm from keratosis pilaris, psoriasis punctata, papular eczema, and lichen ruber?

The distribution and extent of the eruption, the color, the grouping, with usually the presence of pustules and large papules and other concomitant symptoms of syphilis, are points of difference. Pustules never occur in the several diseases named, except in eczema.

Describe the large-papular eruption of syphilis.

The *large-papular syphiloderm* (or *lenticular syphiloderm*) is a common form of cutaneous syphilis, appearing usually in the first six or eight months, and consists of a more or less generalized eruption of pea- to dime-sized or larger, flat, rounded or oval, firmly-seated,

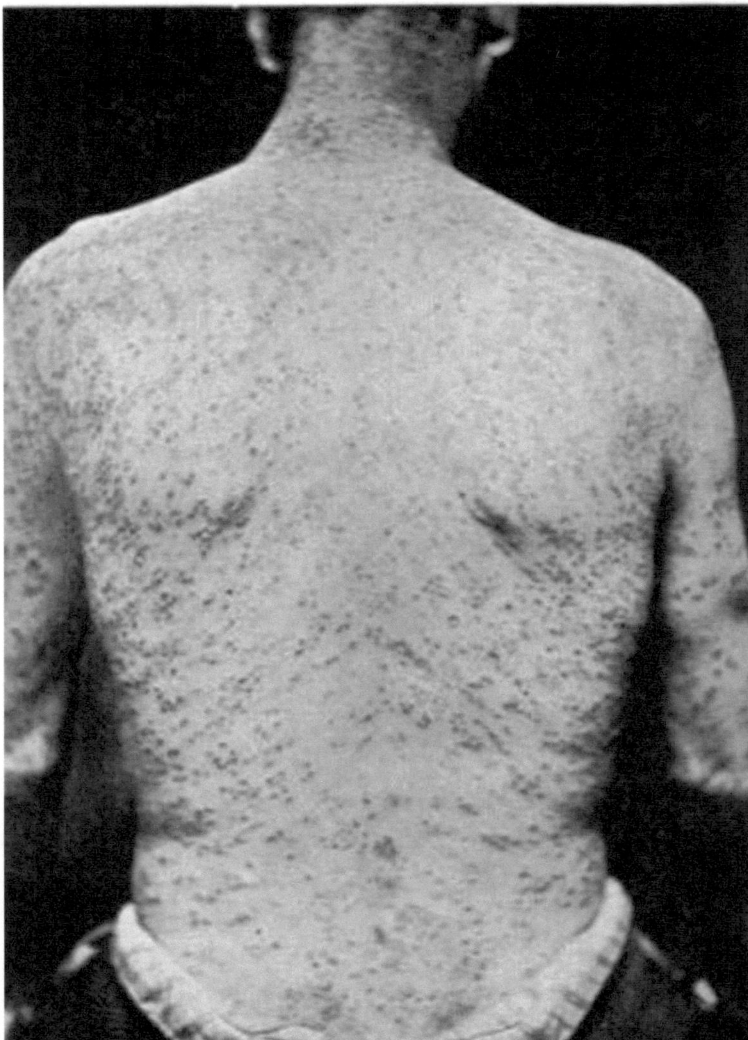

Small-papular Syphiloderm.

[Pg 217]

more or less raised, dull-red papules; with at first a smooth surface, which later usually becomes covered with a film of exfoliating epidermis. The papules, as a rule, develop slowly, remain stationary several weeks or a few months, and then pass away by absorption, leaving slight pigmentation, which gradually fades; or they may undergo certain modifications. In most cases it responds rapidly to treatment.

Fig. 53.

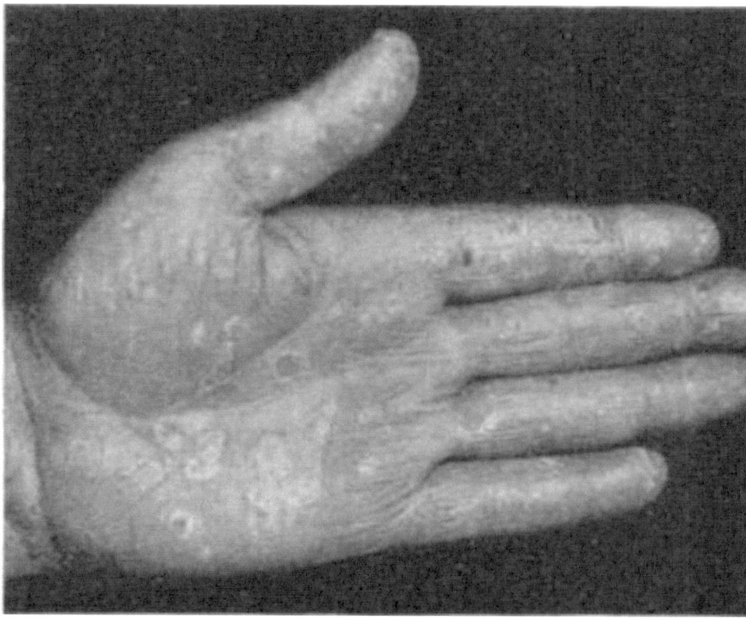

Palmar Syphiloderm.

What modifications do the papules of the large-papular syphiloderm sometimes undergo?

They may change into the moist papule and squamous papule.

Describe the moist papule of syphilis.

The change into the moist papule (also called *mucous patch, flat condyloma*) is not uncommon where opposing surfaces and natural folds of skin are subjected to more or less contact, as about the anus, the scroto-femoral regions, umbilicus, axillæ and beneath the [Pg 218] mammæ. The dry, flat papules gradually become moist and covered with a grayish, sticky, mucoid secretion; several may coalesce and form large, flat patches. They may so remain, or they may become hypertrophic, warty or papillomatous, with more or less crust formation (*vegetating syphiloderm*).

Fig. 54.

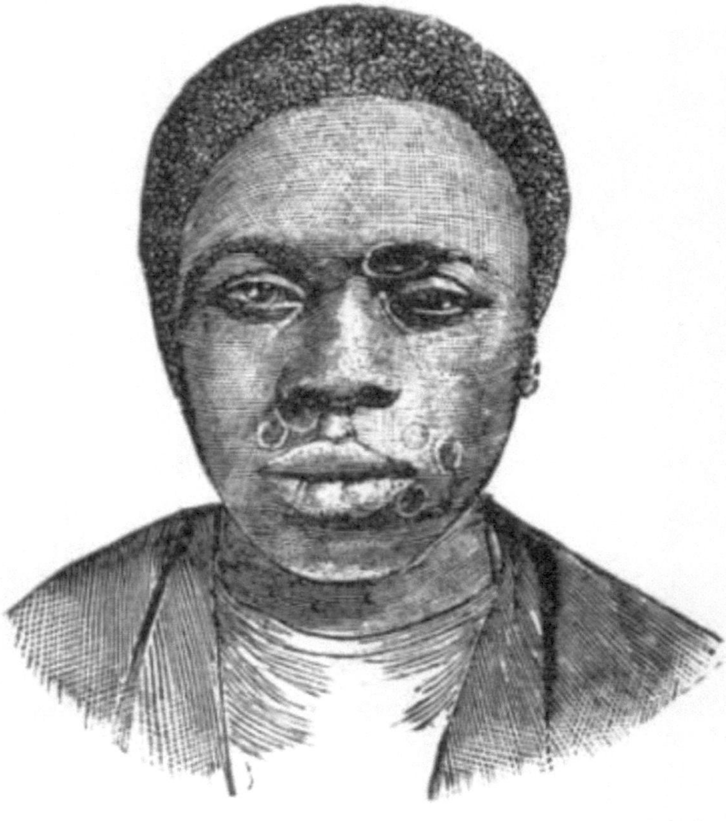

Annular Syphiloderm. (*After I.E. Atkinson.*)

Describe the squamous papule of syphilis.

This tendency of the large-papular eruption to become scaly, when exhibited, is more or less common to all papules, and constitutes the *squamous* or *papulo-squamous syphiloderm* (improperly called *psoriasis syphilitica*). The papules become somewhat flattened and are covered with dry, grayish or dirty-gray, somewhat adherent scales. The scaling, as compared to that of psoriasis, is, as a rule, relatively slight. The eruption may be general, as usually the case in the earlier months of the disease, or it may appear as a relapse or a later manifestation, and be limited in extent.

As a limited eruption it is most frequently seen on the palms and soles — the *palmar and plantar syphiloderm*. Occurring on these parts it is often rebellious to treatment.

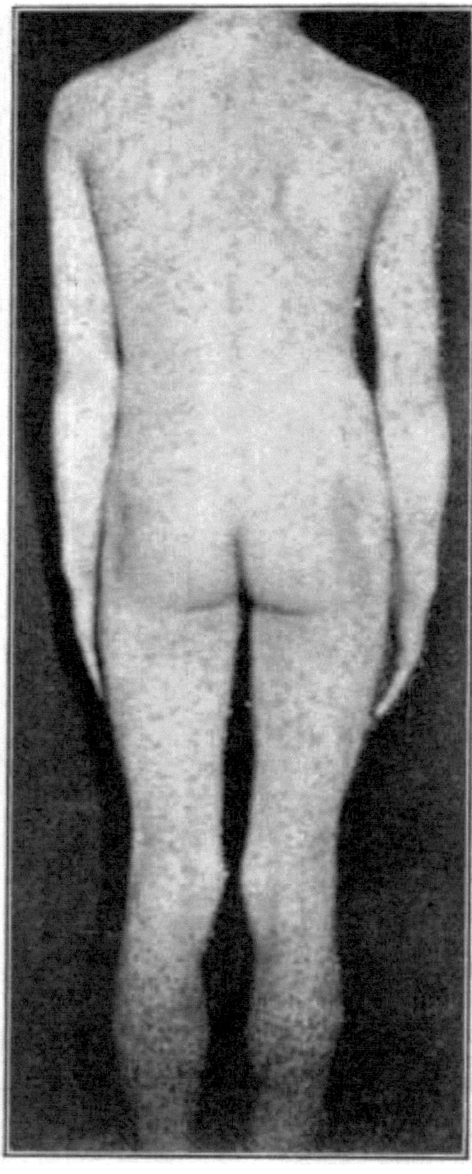

Maculo-papular syphiloderm.

[Pg 219]

How are you to distinguish the papulo-squamous syphiloderm from psoriasis?

In psoriasis the eruption is more inflammatory, and usually bright red; the scales whitish or pearl-colored and, as a rule, abundant. It is generally seen in greater profusion upon certain parts, as, for instance, the extensor surfaces, especially of the elbows and knees. It is not infrequently itchy, and, moreover, presents a different history.

In the syphilitic eruption some of the papules almost invariably remain perfectly free from any tendency to scale formation; there is distinct deposit or infiltration, and the lesions are of a dark, sluggish red or ham tint; and, moreover, concomitant symptoms of syphilis are usually present.

Describe the annular eruption of syphilis.

The *annular syphiloderm* (*circinate syphiloderm*) is observed usually in association with the large-papular eruption, and consists of several or more variously sized, ring-like lesions, with a distinctly elevated solid ridge or wall peripherally and a more or less flattened centre. It is commonly seen about the mouth, forehead and neck. The lesion appears to have its origin from an ordinary, usually scaleless or slightly scaly, large papule, the central portion of which has been incompletely formed or has become sunken and flattened. The manifestation is rare, and is seen most frequently in the negro.

What several varieties of the pustular syphiloderm are met with?

The small acuminated-pustular syphiloderm, the large acuminated-pustular syphiloderm, the small flat-pustular syphiloderm, and the large flat-pustular syphiloderm.

Describe the small acuminated-pustular eruption of syphilis.

The *small acuminated-pustular syphiloderm* (*miliary pustular syphiloderm*) is an early or late secondary eruption, commonly encountered in the first six or eight months of the disease. It consists of a more or less generalized, disseminated or grouped, millet-seed-sized, acuminated pustules, usually seated upon dull-red, papular elevations. The eruption is, as a rule, profuse, and usually involves the hair-follicles. The pustules dry to crusts, which fall off and are often followed by a slight, fringe-like exfoliation [Pg 220] around the base, constituting a grayish ring or collar. Minute pin-point atrophic depressions or stains are left, which gradually become less distinct. Scattered large pustules, and sometimes papules, are not infrequently present.

Describe the large acuminated-pustular eruption of syphilis.

The *large acuminated-pustular syphiloderm* (*acne-form syphiloderm, variola-form syphiloderm*) is a more or less generalized eruption, occurring usually in the first six or eight months of the disease. It consists of small or large pea-sized, disseminated or grouped, acuminated or rounded pustules, resembling the lesions of acne and variola. They develop slowly or rapidly, and at first may appear more or less papular. They dry to somewhat thick crusts, and are seated upon superficially ulcerated bases.

It pursues, as a rule, a comparatively rapid and benign course. In relapses the eruption is usually more or less localized.

How would you distinguish the large acuminated-pustular syphiloderm from acne and variola?

In acne the usual limitation of the lesions to the face or face and shoulders, the origin, more rapid formation and evolution of the individual lesions, and the chronic character of the disease, are usually distinctive points.

In variola, the intensity of the general symptoms, the shot-like beginning of the lesions, their course, the umbilication, and the definite duration, are to be considered.

The presence or absence of other symptoms of syphilis has, in obscure cases, an important diagnostic bearing.

Describe the small flat-pustular eruption of syphilis.

The *small flat-pustular syphiloderm* (*impetigo-form syphiloderm*) consists of a more or less generalized, pea-sized, flat or raised, discrete, irregularly-grouped, or in places confluent, pustules, appearing usually in the first year of the disease. The pustules dry rapidly to yellow, greenish-yellow, or brownish, more or less adherent, thick, uneven, somewhat granular crusts, beneath which there may be superficial or deep ulceration; where the lesions are confluent a continuous sheet of crusting forms. The eruption is often scanty. It is most frequently observed about the nose, mouth, hairy parts of the face and [Pg 221] scalp, and about the genitalia, frequently in association with papules on other parts.

Are you likely to mistake the small flat-pustular syphiloderm for any other eruption?

Scarcely; but when upon the scalp, it may bear rough resemblance to pustular eczema, but the erosion or ulceration will serve to differentiate. Moreover, concomitant symptoms of syphilis are to be looked for.

Describe the large flat-pustular eruption of syphilis.

The *large flat-pustular syphiloderm* (*ecthyma-form syphiloderm*) consists of a more or less generalized, scattered eruption, of large pea- or dime-sized, flat pustules. They dry rapidly to crusts. The bases of the lesions are a deep-red or copper color. Two types of the eruption are met with.

In one type—the superficial variety—the crust is flat, rounded or ovalish, of a yellowish-brown or dark-brown color, and seated upon a superficial erosion or ulcer. The lesions are usually numerous, and most abundant on the back, shoulders and extremities. It appears, as a rule, within the first year, and generally runs a benign course.

Fig. 55.

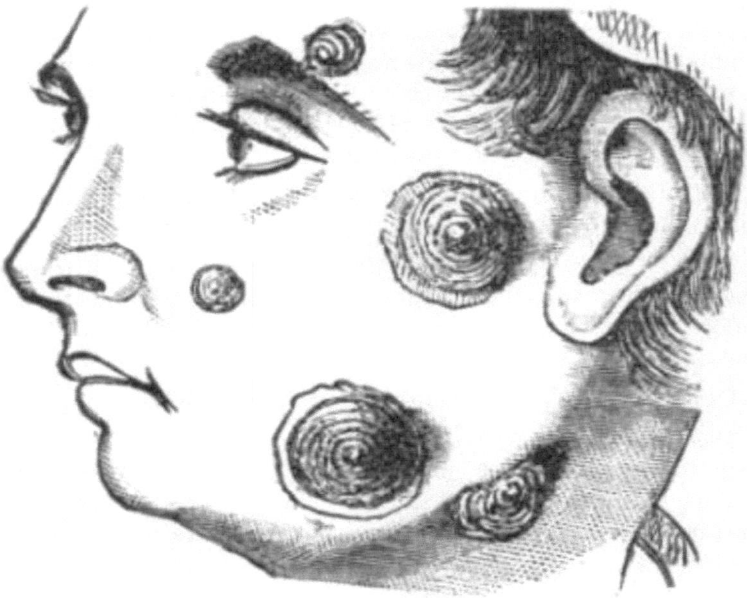

Rupia. (*After Tilbury Fox.*)

[Pg 222] In the other type—the deep variety—the crust is greenish or blackish, is raised and more bulky, often conical and stratified, like an oyster shell—*rupia*; beneath the crusts may be seen rounded or irregular-shaped ulcers, having a greenish-yellow, puriform secretion. It is usually a late and malignant manifestation.

How would you differentiate the large flat-pustular syphiloderm from ecthyma?

The syphilitic lesions are more numerous, are scattered, are attended with superficial or deep ulceration, and followed by more or less scar-formation. Moreover, the history, and presence or absence of other symptoms of syphilis have an important diagnostic value.

Fig. 56.

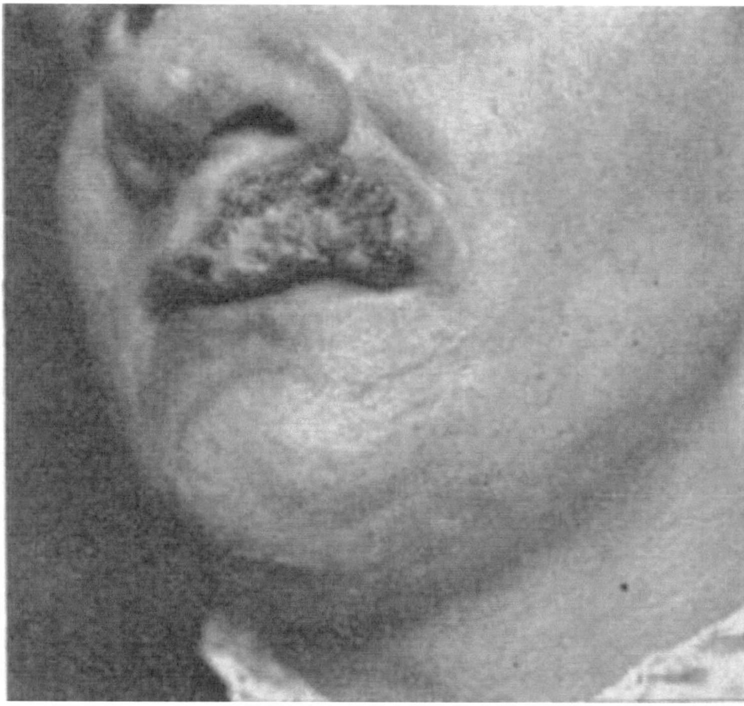

Ulcerating Tubercular Syphiloderm.

Describe the bullous eruption of syphilis.

The *bullous syphiloderm*, (of acquired syphilis) is a rare and usually late eruption, appearing in the form of discrete, disseminated, rounded or ovalish, pea- to walnut-sized, partially or fully distended, blebs. The serous contents soon become cloudy and puriform. In some cases the lesions are distinctly pustular from the beginning. [Pg 223] The crust, which soon forms, is of a yellowish-brown or dark green color, and may be thick and stratified (*rupia*), as in the deep variety of the large flat-pustular syphiloderm. The erosions or ulcers beneath the crusts secrete a greenish-yellow fluid. It is a malignant type of eruption, and is usually seen in broken-down subjects.

It is not an uncommon manifestation of hereditary syphilis (*q. v.*) in the newborn.

Fig. 57.

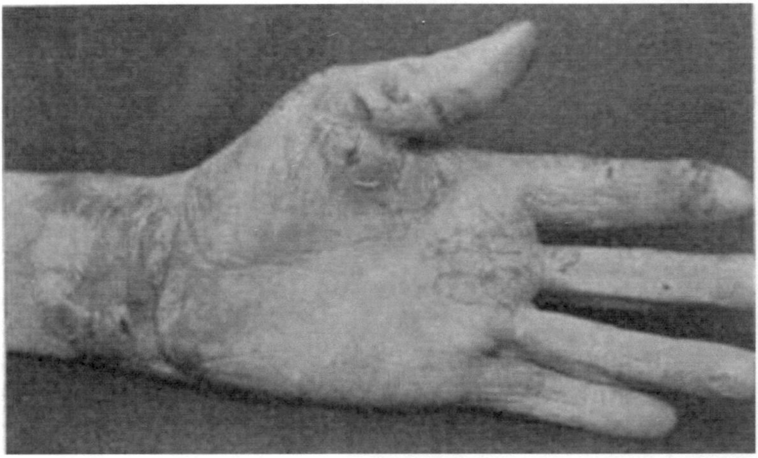

Tubercular Syphiloderm.

How is the bullous syphiloderm to be differentiated from other pemphigoid eruptions?

By the gravity of the disease, the accompanying ulceration, the course and history; and by other evidences, past or present, of syphilis.

Describe the tubercular eruption of syphilis.

The *tubercular syphiloderm* (*syphiloderma tuberculosum*) may exceptionally occur within the first year as a more or less generalized eruption. As a rule, however, it is a late manifestation, at times appearing many years after the initial lesion; is limited in extent, and shows a decided tendency to occur in groups, often forming [Pg 224] segments of circles and circular areas, clearing in the centre and spreading peripherally.

It consists (as a late, limited manifestation) of several or more firm, circumscribed, deeply-seated, smooth, glistening or slightly scaly elevations; rounded or acuminated in shape, of a yellowish-red, brownish-red or coppery color and usually of the size of small or large peas. Several groups may coalesce, and a serpiginous tract result (*serpiginous tubercular syphiloderm*). The lesions develop slowly, and are sluggish in their course, remaining, at times, for weeks or months, with but little change. As a rule, however, they terminate sooner or later, either by absorption, leaving a more or less permanent pigment stain with or without slight atrophy (*non-ulcerating tubercular syphiloderm*), or by ulceration (*ulcerating tubercular syphiloderm*).

Describe the ulcerating tubercular syphiloderm.

Fig. 58.

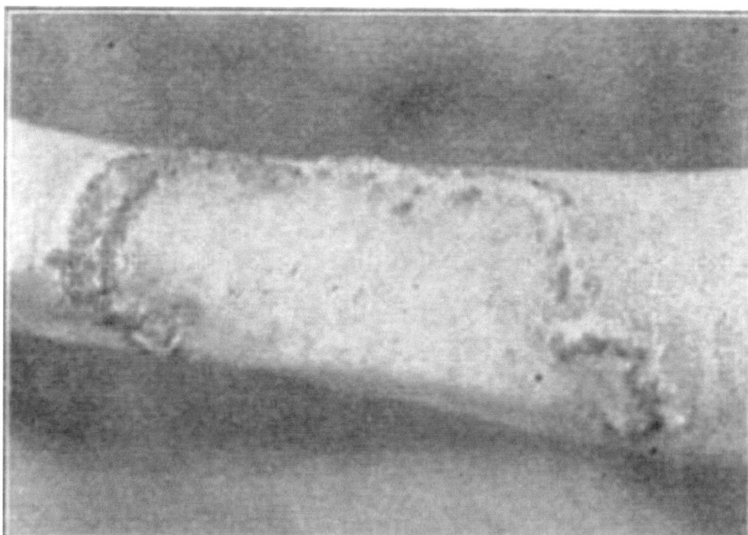

Ulcerating Tubercular Syphiloderm.

The ulceration may be superficial or deep in character, and involve several or all of the lesions forming the group. The patch may consist, therefore, of small, discrete, punched-out ulcers, or of one or more continuous ulcers, segmented, crescentic or serpiginous in shape. They are covered with a gummy, grayish-yellow deposit or they may be crusted. As the ulcerative changes take place, new

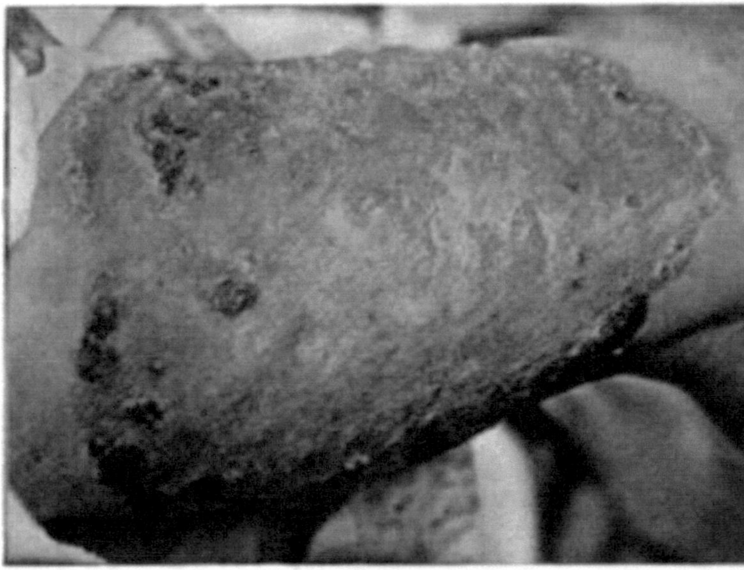

Tubercular Syphiloderm.

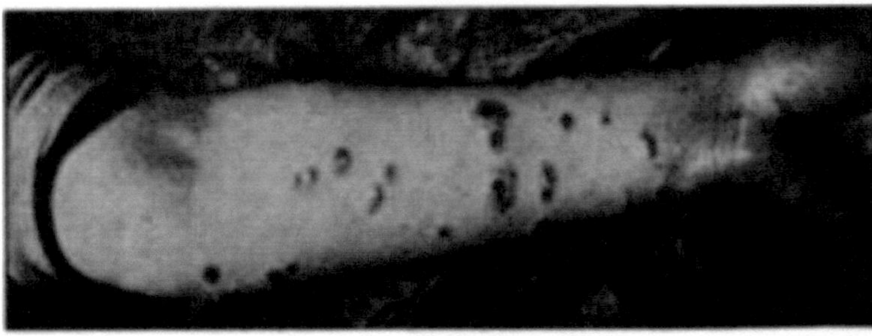

Large-pustular Syphiloderm.

[Pg 225]

lesions, especially about the periphery of the group or patch, may appear from time to time.

In some instances, more especially about the scalp, the surface of the ulcerations becomes papillary or wart-like, with an offensive, yellowish, puriform secretion (*syphilis cutanea papillomatosa*).

From what diseases is the tubercular syphiloderm to be differentiated?

From tubercular leprosy, epithelioma and lupus vulgaris, especially the last-named.

What are the chief diagnostic characters of the tubercular syphiloderm?

The tendency to form segments, crescents and circles, the color, the pigmentation and ulceration, the history, and not infrequently marks or scars of former eruptions.

Fig. 59.

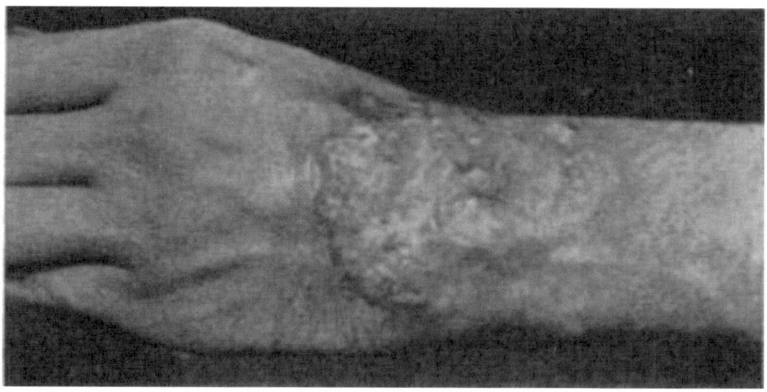

Tubercular Syphiloderm.

Describe the gummatous eruption of syphilis.

The *gummatous syphiloderm* (*syphiloderma gummatosum, gumma, syphiloma*) is usually a late manifestation, showing itself as one, several or more painless or slightly painful, rounded or flat, more or less circumscribed tumors; they are slightly raised, moderately firm, and have their seat in the subcutaneous tissue. They tend to break down and ulcerate. [Pg 226] The lesion begins usually as a pea-sized deposit or infiltration, and grows slowly or rapidly; when fully developed it may be the size of a walnut, or even larger. The overlying skin becomes gradually reddish. At first firm, it is later soft and doughy. It may, even when well advanced, disappear by absorption, but usually tends to break down, terminating in a small or large, deep, punched-out ulcer.

Fig. 60.

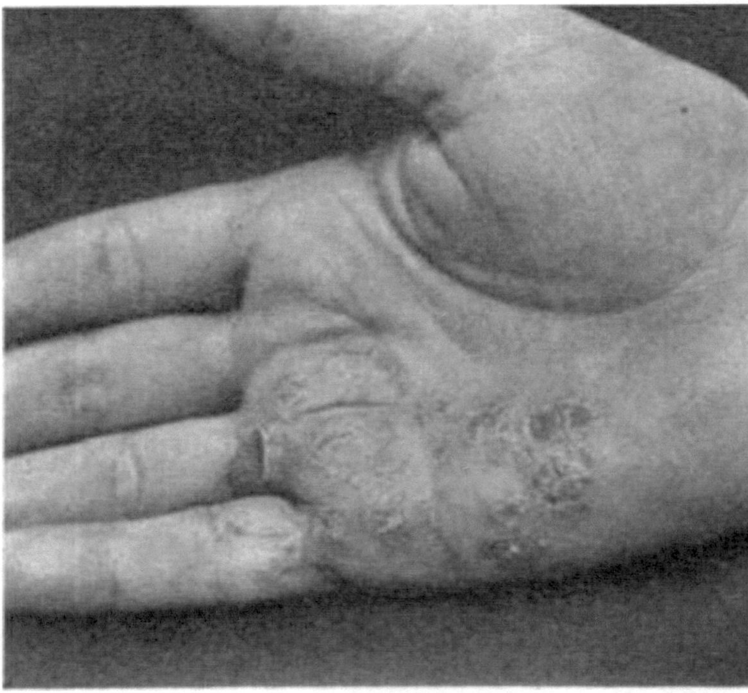

Tubercular Syphiloderm.

Does the gummatous syphiloderm invariably appear as a rounded well-defined tumor?

No. Exceptionally, instead of a well-defined tumor, it may appear as a more or less diffused patch of infiltration, leading eventually to extensive superficial or deep ulceration.

From what formations is the gummatous syphiloderm to be differentiated?

From furuncle, abscess, and sebaceous, fatty and fibroid tumors. [Pg 227] Attention to the origin, course, and behavior of the lesion, together with a history, must all be considered in doubtful cases.

Fig. 61.

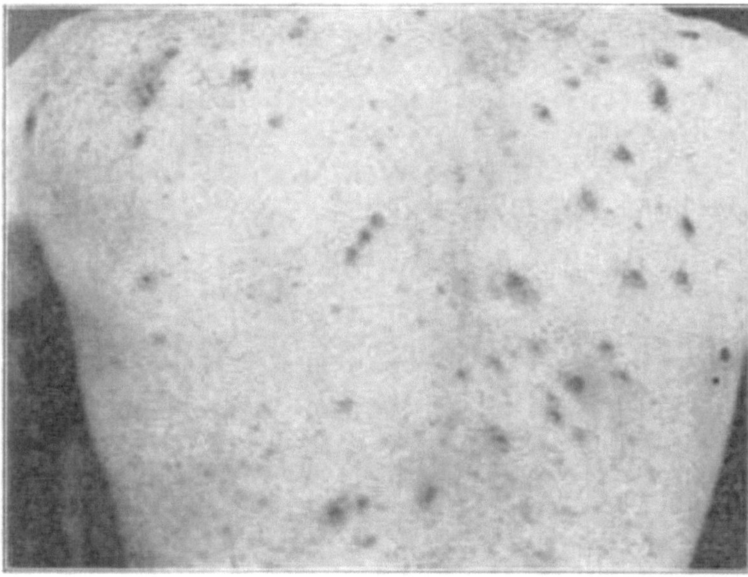

Large Pustular Syphiloderm.

What is to be said in regard to the character and time of appearance of the cutaneous manifestations of hereditary syphilis?

In a great measure the cutaneous manifestations of hereditary syphilis are essentially the same as observed in acquired syphilis. They are usually noted to occur within the first three months of extra-uterine life. The macular, papular, and bullous eruptions are most common.

Describe these several cutaneous manifestations of hereditary syphilis.

The *macular* (erythematous) eruption begins as large or small, bright- or dark-red macules, later presenting a ham or café-au-lait appearance. At first they disappear upon pressure. The lesions are more or less numerous, usually become confluent, especially about the folds of the neck, about the genitalia and buttocks; in these regions resembling somewhat erythema intertrigo.

The *papular* eruption is observed in conjunction with the [Pg 228] erythematous manifestation, or it occurs alone. The lesions are but slightly elevated, and seem to partake of the nature of both macules and papules. They are usually discrete, and rarely abundant; they may become decked with a film-like scale, and at the various points of junction of skin and mucous membrane, and in the folds, they become abraded and macerated, developing into *moist papules*.

The *bullous* eruption consists of variously-sized, more or less purulent blebs, and is usually met with at or immediately following birth. It is most abundant about the hands and feet. Macules and papules are often interspersed. There may be superficial or deep ulceration underlying the bullæ.

What other symptoms in addition to the cutaneous manifestations are noted in hereditary syphilis in the newborn?

Mucous patches, and sometimes ulcers, in the mouth and throat; hoarseness, as shown by the peculiar cry, and indicating involvement of the larynx; snuffles, a sallow and dirty appearance of the skin, loss of flesh and often a shriveled or senile look.

What is the pathology of cutaneous syphilis?

The syphilitic deposit consists of round-cell infiltration. The mucous layer, the corium, and in the deep lesions the subcutaneous connective tissues also, are involved in the process. The infiltration disappears by absorption or ulceration. The factor now believed to be responsible for the disease and the pathological changes is the Spirochæta pallida, discovered by Schaudinn and Hoffmann, and usually found in numbers in the tissues.

Give the prognosis of cutaneous syphilis.

In *acquired syphilis*, favorable; sooner or later, unless the whole system is so profoundly affected by the syphilitic poison that a fatal ending ensues, the cutaneous manifestations disappear, either spontaneously or as the result of treatment. The earlier eruptions will often pass away without medication, but treatment is of material aid in moderating their severity and hastening their disappearance, and is to be looked upon as essential; in the late syphilodermata treatment is indispensable. In the large pustular, the tubercular and gummatous lesions, considerable destruction of tissue may take place, and in consequence scarring result. Ill-health from any cause predisposes to a relapse, and also adds to the gravity of the case.

In *hereditary infantile syphilis*, the prognosis is always uncertain: [Pg 229] the more distant from the time of birth the manifestations appear the more favorable usually is the outcome.

How is cutaneous syphilis to be treated?

Always with constitutional remedies; and in the graver eruptions, and especially in those more or less limited, with local applications also.

What constitutional and local remedies are commonly employed in cutaneous syphilis?

Constitutional Remedies.—Mercury and potassium iodide; tonics and nutrients are necessary in some cases.

Local Remedies.—Mercurial ointments, lotions and baths, and iodol in ointment or in (and also calomel) powder form.

Give the constitutional treatment of the earlier, or secondary, eruptions of syphilis.

In secondary or early eruptions mercury alone in almost every case; with tonics, if called for. If mercury is contraindicated (extremely rare), potassium iodide may be substituted.

How is mercury usually administered in the eruptions of secondary syphilis?

By the mouth, chiefly as the protiodide, calomel and blue mass, in dosage just short of mild physiological action; by *inunction*, in the form of blue ointment; by *hypodermic injection*, usually as corrosive sublimate solution. The method by *fumigation*, with calomel or bisulphuret, is now rarely employed.

The method by the mouth is the common one, and it is only in rare instances that any other method is necessary or advisable.

What local applications are usually advised in the eruptions of secondary syphilis?

If the eruption is extensive, and more especially in the pustular types, baths of corrosive sublimate (ʒii-ʒiv] to Cong. xxx) may be used; and ointment of ammoniated mercury, twenty to sixty grains to the ounce, blue ointment, and the ten per cent. oleate of mercury alone or with an equal quantity of any ointment base.

The same applications or a dusting powder of calomel may also be used on moist papules. [Pg 230]

How long is mercury to be actively continued in cases of early (secondary) syphilis?

Until one or two months after all manifestations (cutaneous or other) have disappeared, and then, as a general rule, continued, as a small daily dose (about one-quarter to one-third of that prescribed during the active treatment) for a period of two or three months; then another cycle of the active dosage for a period of four to six weeks; then a resumption of the smaller daily dose for another two or three months; and so on, for a period of at least two years.

(Almost all authorities are agreed as to the importance of prolonged treatment, but differ somewhat on the question of intermittent or uninterrupted administration.)

Give the constitutional treatment of the late, or localized, syphilodermata.

Mercury always, usually in small or moderate dosage, as the biniodide or corrosive chloride, and potassium iodide; the latter in dose varying from two grains to two drachms or more, t.d., depending upon its action and the urgency of the case.

How long is constitutional treatment to be continued in cases of the late syphilodermata?

Actively for several weeks after the disappearance of all symptoms, and then (especially the mercury) continued in smaller dosage (about one-third) for several months longer.

What applications are usually advised in the late, or localized, syphilodermata?

Ointment of ammoniated mercury, twenty to sixty grains to the ounce; oleate of mercury, five to ten per cent. strength; mercurial plaster, full strength or weakened with lard or petrolatum; a two to twenty per cent. ointment of iodol; resorcin, twenty to sixty grains to the ounce of ointment base; and lotions of corrosive sublimate, one-half to three grains to the ounce.

The following is valuable in offensive and obstinate ulcerations:—

℞ Hydrarg. chlorid. corros., ... gr. iv-gr. viij Ac. carbolici, ... gr. x-xx Alcoholis, ... fʒiv Glycerinæ, ... fʒj Aquæ, ... q.s. ad. .... ℥iv. M.

[Pg 231] Ointments are to be rubbed in or applied as a plaster; lotions, employed chiefly in ulcers and ulcerations, are to be thoroughly dabbed on, and usually supplemented by the application of an ointment. Iodol may also be applied to ulcers as a dusting-powder, usually mixed with one to several parts of zinc oxide or boric acid.

Give the treatment of hereditary infantile syphilis.

It is essentially the same (but much smaller dosage) as employed in acquired syphilis. Attention to proper feeding and hygiene is of first importance.

Mercury may be given by the mouth, as mercury with chalk (gr. ss-gr. ij, t.d.); as calomel (gr. 1/20-gr. 1/6, t.d.); and as a solution of corrosive sublimate (gr. ss-℥vj, ʒj, t.d.). If mercury is not well borne by the stomach, it may be administered by inunction; for this purpose, blue ointment is mixed with one or two parts of lard and spread (about a drachm) upon an abdominal bandage and applied, being renewed daily. Treatment by means of baths (gr. x-xxx to the bath) of corrosive sublimate is, at times, a serviceable method.

Potassium iodide, if exceptionally deemed preferable, may be given in the dose of a fractional part of a grain to two or three grains three times daily.

What local measures are to be advised in cutaneous syphilis of the newborn?

If demanded, applications similar to those employed in eruptions of acquired syphilis, but not more than one-third to one-half the strength.

Lepra.

(*Synonyms:* Leprosy; Elephantiasis Græcorum.)

What do you understand by leprosy?

Lepra, or leprosy, is an endemic, chronic, malignant constitutional disease, characterized by alterations in the cutaneous, nerve, and bone structures; varying in its morbid manifestations according to whether the skin, nerves or other tissues are predominantly involved.

What is the nature of the premonitory symptoms of leprosy?

In some instances the active manifestations appear without [Pg 232] premonition, but in the majority of cases symptoms, slight or severe in character, pointing toward profound constitutional disturbance, such as mental depression, malaise, chills, febrile attacks, digestive derangements and bone pains, are noticed for weeks, months, or several years preceding the outbreak.

What several varieties of leprosy are observed?

Two definite forms are usually described—the tubercular and the anæsthetic. A sharp division-line cannot, however, always be drawn; not infrequently the manifestations are of a mixed type, or one form may pass into or gradually present symptoms of the other.

Fig. 62.

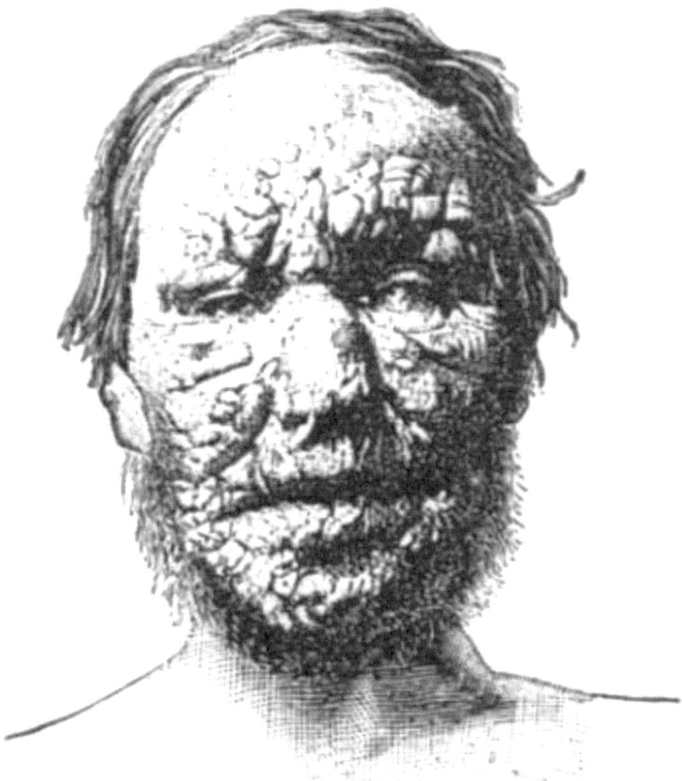

Tubercular Leprosy. (*After Stoddard.*)

Describe the symptoms of tubercular leprosy.

The formation of tubercles and tubercular masses of infiltration, usually of a yellowish-brown color, with subsequent ulceration, constitute the important cutaneous symptoms. Along with, or preceding these characteristic lesions, blebs and more or less infiltrated, hyperæsthetic or anæsthetic, pinkish, reddish or pale-yellowish [Pg 233] macules make their appearance from time to time; subsequently fading away or remaining permanently (*lepra maculosa*).

When well advanced, the tubercular or nodular masses give rise to great deformity; the face, a favorite locality, becomes more or less leonine in appearance (*leontiasis*). The tubercles persist almost indefinitely without material change, or undergo absorption or ulceration; this last takes place most commonly about the fingers and toes. The mucous membrane of the mouth, pharynx and other parts may also become involved.

Fig. 63.

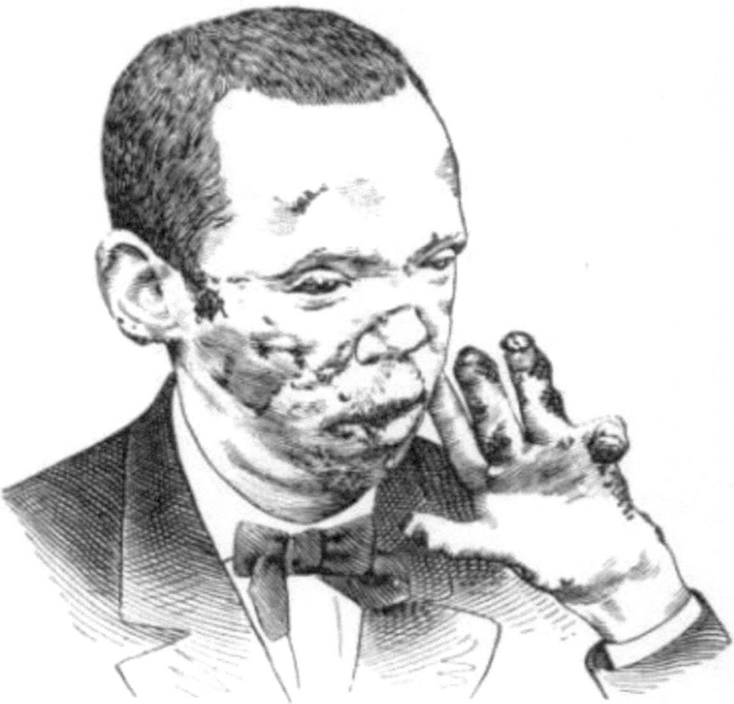

Anæsthetic Leprosy.

Describe the symptoms of anæsthetic leprosy.

Following or along with precursory symptoms denoting general systemic disturbance, or independently of any prodromal indications, a hyperæsthetic condition, in localized areas or more or less general, is observed. Lancinating pains along the nerves and an irregular [Pg 234] pemphigoid eruption are also commonly noted. There soon follows the special eruption, coming out from time to time, and consisting of several or more, usually non-elevated, well-defined, pale-yellowish patches, one or two inches in diameter. As a rule, they are at first neither hyperæsthetic nor anæsthetic, but may be the seat of slight burning or itching. They spread peripherally, and tend to clear in the centre. The patches eventually become markedly anæsthetic, and the overlying skin, and the skin on other parts as well, becomes atrophic and of a brownish or yellowish color. The subcutaneous tissues, muscle, hair and nails undergo atrophic or degenerative changes, and these changes are especially noted about the hands and feet. These parts become crooked, the bone tissues are involved, the phalanges dropping off or disappearing by disintegration or absorption (*lepra mutilans*). Sooner or later various paralytic symptoms, showing more active involvement of the nerve trunks, present themselves.

State the cause of leprosy.

Present knowledge points to a peculiar bacillus as the active factor, while climate, soil, heredity, food and habits exert a predisposing influence.

Is leprosy contagious?

The consensus of opinion points to the acceptance of the possible contagiousness of leprosy; probably by inoculation, but only under certain unknown favoring conditions.

What are the pathological changes?

The lesions consist essentially of a new growth, made up of numerous small, more or less aggregated round cells, beginning in the walls of the bloodvessels. In this way the tubercular masses and various other lesions are formed. As yet, positive involvement ot the central nervous system has not been shown, but some of the nerve trunks are found to be inflamed and swollen, with a tendency toward hardening.

What several diseases are to be eliminated in the diagnosis of leprosy?

Syphilis, morphœa, vitiligo, lupus, and syringomyelia.

When well advanced, the aggregate symptoms of leprosy form a [Pg 235] picture which can scarcely be confused with that of any other disease. In doubtful cases microscopical examinations of the involved tissues, for the bacilli, should be made.

State the prognosis of leprosy.

Unfavorable; a fatal termination is the rule, but may not be reached for a number of years. The tubercular form is the most grave, the mixed variety next, and the anæsthetic the least. Patients are not infrequently carried off by intercurrent disease. Proper management will often delay the fatal ending, and exceptionally, in the anæsthetic variety, stay the progress of the disease.

What is the treatment of leprosy?

Hygienic measures are important. Chaulmoogra oil and gurjun oil internally and externally are in some instances of service. Strychnia alone, or with either of these oils, is ofttimes beneficial. Ichthyol internally, and external applications of the same drug, and of resorcin, chrysarobin, and pyrogallic acid, have been extolled. Change of climate, especially to a region where the disease does not prevail, is often of great advantage.

Pellagra.

(*Synonym:* Lombardian Leprosy.)

Describe pellagra.

Pellagra is a slow but usually progressive disease occurring chiefly in Italy, due, it is thought, to the continued ingestion of decomposed or fermented maize. It is characterized by cutaneous symptoms, at first upon exposed parts, of an erythematous, desquamative, vesicular and bullous character, and by general constitutional disturbance of a markedly neurotic type. A fatal ending, if the disease is at all severe or advanced, is to be expected.

Treatment is based upon general principles. [Pg 236]

Epithelioma.

(*Synonyms:* Skin Cancer; Epithelial Cancer; Carcinoma Epitheliale.)

What several varieties of epithelioma are met with?

Three—the superficial, the deep-seated, and the papillomatous.

Describe the clinical appearances and course of the superficial variety of epithelioma.

The superficial, or flat variety (*rodent ulcer*), begins, usually on the face, as a minute, firm, reddish or yellowish tubercle, as an

Fig. 64.

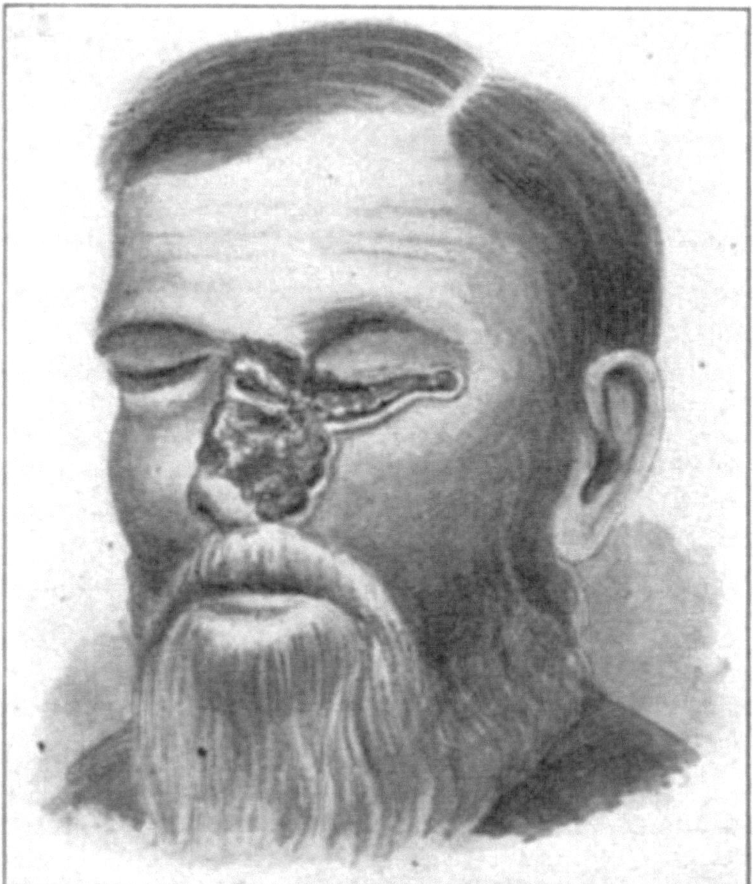

Epithelioma. (*After D. Lewis.*)

aggregation of such, as a warty excrescence, or as a localized degenerative seborrhœic patch. The latter lesion (known also as keratosis senilis, old-age atrophic patches), consisting of a yellowish or yellowish-brown greasy or hardened scurfy spot or patch is quite frequently the starting-point of epithelial growths. Sooner or later, commonly after months or several years, the surface becomes slightly excoriated, and an insignificant, yellowish or brownish crust is formed. The excoriation gradually develops into superficial [Pg 237] ulceration, and the diseased area becomes slowly larger and larger. New lesions may continue, from time to time, to appear about the edges and go through the same changes.

The ulcer has usually an uneven surface, secretes a thin, scanty, viscid fluid, which dries to a firm, adherent crust. It is usually defined against the healthy skin by a slightly elevated, hard, roll-like, waxy-looking border. In rare instances there is a disposition, at points, to spontaneous involution and scar formation; as a rule, however, the ulcerative action slowly progresses.

The general health is unimpaired, the neighboring lymphatic glands are not involved, and the local condition, beyond the disfigurement, gives rise to little trouble, unless, as occasionally happens, it passes into the more malignant, deep-seated variety.

Describe the clinical appearances and course of the deep-seated variety of epithelioma.

The deep-seated variety starts from the superficial form, or it begins as a tubercle or nodule in the skin. When typically developed, a reddish, shining tubercle or nodule, or area of infiltration, forms in the skin or subcutaneous tissue. In the course of weeks or months superficial or deep-seated ulceration takes place; the ulcer having hardened, and, as a rule, everted edges. The surface is reddish and granular, and secretes an ichorous discharge. The infiltration spreads, the ulcer enlarges both peripherally and in depth— muscle, cartilage and bone often becoming invaded. The neighboring lymphatic gland may become implicated, pains of a burning or neuralgic type are experienced, and from septicæmia, marasmus, or involvement of vital parts, death eventually ensues.

Describe the clinical appearances and course of the papillomatous variety of epithelioma.

The papillomatous type usually arises from the superficial or deep-seated variety, or it may begin as a papillary or warty growth. When fully developed, it presents an ulcerated, fissured and papillomatous surface, with an ichorous discharge which dries to crusts. It is slowly progressive, and sooner or later may develop a malignant tendency.

Upon what parts is epithelioma commonly observed?

About the face, especially the nose, eyelids and lips; and also about the genitalia. It may involve any part. [Pg 238]

At what age is epithelioma usually noted?

It is essentially a disease of middle and late life, although it is exceptionally met with in the young.

What is the cause of epithelioma?

The etiology is obscure. It is not, as a rule, inherited. Any locally irritated tissue may be the starting point of the disease.

State the pathology.

The process consists in the proliferation of epithelial cells from the mucous layer; the cell-growth takes place downward, in the form of finger-like prolongations or columns, or it may spread out laterally, so as to form rounded masses, the centres of which usually undergo horny transformation, resulting in the formation of onion-like bodies, the so-called cell-nests or globes. The rapid cell-growth requires increased nutriment, and hence the bloodvessels become enlarged; moreover, the pressure of the cell-masses gives rise to irritation and inflammation, with corresponding serous and round-cell infiltration.

How would you distinguish epithelioma from syphilitic ulceration, wart, and lupus vulgaris?

From syphilis it is to be differentiated by the history, duration, character of the base and edges, its comparative slow progress, its usually slight, viscid discharge, often streaked with blood, and, if necessary, by the therapeutic test.

Wart or warty growths are to be differentiated by attention to their history and course. Long-continued observation may be necessary before a positive opinion is warrantable. The appearance of any tendency to crusting, to break down or ulcerate is significant of epitheliomatous degeneration.

In lupus vulgaris the deposits are peculiar and multiple, the ulcerations are of different character, the tendency to scar-formation constant; and, with few exceptions, it has, moreover, its beginning in childhood or early adult life.

What factors are to be considered in giving a prognosis in epithelioma?

The variety, extent, and rapidity of the process. The superficial form may exist for years, and give rise to no alarm; whereas the [Pg 239] deeper-seated varieties are always to be viewed as serious, and are, indeed, often fatal. Involving the genitalia, its course is often strikingly rapid. Relapses, after removal, are not uncommon.

What is the special object in view in the treatment of epithelioma?

Thorough destruction or removal of the epitheliomatous tissue.

How is the destruction or removal of the epitheliomatous tissue effected?

By the use of such caustics as caustic potash, chloride-of-zinc paste, pyrogallic acid, arsenic, and the galvano-cautery; and by operative measures, such as excision and erasion with the dermal curette, and by the *x*-ray. (See treatment of lupus vulgaris.)

In small lesions the use of an arsenical paste is a most admirable method of treatment, although somewhat painful. The paste is made of one part powdered acacia and one to two parts arsenious acid; at the time of application sufficient water is added to make a paste. This is applied thickly, and a piece of lint superimposed. A good deal of pain and inflammatory swelling ensue; at the end of twenty-four hours the part is poulticed till the slough comes away; the ulcer is then treated as a simple ulcer, under which healing takes place. Occasionally a second application is found necessary.

Upon the whole, the best method in the average case is to curette thoroughly, and supplement with momentary cauterization, with caustic potash, or with several days' use of the pyrogallic acid ointment. During the healing process, short exposures to the Röntgen ray—about every three to five days—is good practice.

The degenerative changes in the beginning of scurfy, seborrhœic spots or patches seen in old people can frequently be lessened or wholly stopped by the daily application of an ointment containing 5 to 10 per cent. of sulphur and 2 to 5 per cent. of salicylic acid.

What can be said of the value of the x-ray in epithelioma?

The *x*-ray method is now much in vogue, and proves curative in many superficial cases, and of benefit in some of the deeper-seated varieties. In most cases it must be pushed to the point of producing a mild *x*-ray erythema; and in some instances benefit or cure only [Pg 240] occurs after more active exposure, sufficient to cause an *x*-ray burn of the second degree. The method is not attended with much risk if properly used. The healthy parts should be protected by lead-foil. Exposure should be two to five times weekly, at a distance of three to eight inches, and from five to twenty minutes, employing a tube of medium vacuum. Unfortunately the method is usually slow. The radium treatment is essentially similar to that by the *x*-ray.

The much better plan, as already intimated, is to employ one of the several operative or caustic methods, and supplementing, while healing, with the *x*-ray.

Paget's Disease of the Nipple.

(*Synonyms:* Malignant Papillary Dermatitis; Paget's Disease.)

What do you understand by Paget's disease of the nipple?

Paget's disease is a rare, inflammatory-looking, malignant disease of the nipple and areola in women, usually of advancing years, eventually terminating in cancerous involvement of the entire gland.

Describe the symptoms of Paget's disease.

The first symptoms, which usually last for months or years, are apparently eczematous, accompanied with more or less burning, itching and tingling. Gradually, the diseased area, which is sharply-defined, and feels like a thin layer of indurated tissue, presents a florid, intensely red, very finely-granular, raw surface, attended with a more or less copious viscid exudation. Sooner or later retraction and destruction of the nipple, followed by gradual scirrhous involvement of the whole breast, takes place.

What is the pathology of Paget's disease?

Although it was thought at one time to be a cancerous disease resulting from a continued eczematous inflammation of the parts, there is now but little doubt that it is of malignant nature from the earliest stages. The psorosperm-like bodies found, to the presence of which the disease has by some authorities been attributed (psorospermosis), are now known to be merely changed and [Pg 241] degenerated epithelia. The morbid changes consist of an inflammation of the papillary region of the derma, leading to œdema and vacuolation of the constituent cells of the epidermis, followed by their complete destruction in places and their abnormal proliferation in others (Fordyce).

State the diagnostic features of Paget's disease.

The age of the patient; the sharp limitation; the well-defined, indurated film of infiltration; the peculiar, red, raw, granulating appearance; and, later, the retraction of the nipple; and, finally, the involvement of the deeper parts.

What is the prognosis?

If the disease is recognized early, and properly treated, a cure may be anticipated; later the outlook is that of scirrhus of the breast.

What is the treatment of Paget's disease?

Thorough cauterization by means of caustic potash or the galvano-cautery; or, its extirpation by means of the curette or excision. After extirpation or cauterization, supplementary treatment by the *x*-ray is advisable as an additional measure of precaution against relapse.

Until the diagnosis is thoroughly established, soothing applications, such as are employed in acute eczema, are to be advised.

Sarcoma.

(*Synonyms:* Sarcoma Cutis; Sarcoma of the Skin.)

Describe the several varieties of sarcoma.

Sarcoma of the skin is a more or less malignant new growth, of rapid or slow progress, characterized by the appearance of single or multiple, variously-shaped, discrete, non-pigmented or pigmented tubercles or tumors, of size varying from that of a shot to a hazelnut or larger. As a rule the growths are smooth, firm and elastic, somewhat painful upon pressure, and exhibit a tendency to ulcerate. The overlying skin is at first normal and somewhat movable, but as the growths approach the surface it becomes reddened and adherent; [Pg 242] or, if the disease is of the pigmented variety, it acquires a bluish-black color. It is now generally believed that the most of the pigmented cases formerly thought to be of sarcomatous nature are really carcinomatous in character.

The multiple pigmented sarcoma (*melano-sarcoma*) appears first, usually on the soles and dorsal surfaces of the feet, and later on the hands. There is more or less diffuse thickening of the integument. The lesions themselves manifest a disposition to bleed.

State the prognosis and treatment of sarcoma.

The disease is always more or less malignant and, as a rule, sooner or later a fatal termination takes place. It is usually slow in its course.

Excision or extirpation, *x*-ray exposures, and the administration of arsenic in increasing dosage (preferably by hypodermic injection) now are generally considered the most promising in this usually hopeless malady.

Granuloma Fungoides.

Describe granuloma fungoides.

A rare form of disease, heretofore looked upon as sarcomatous, but now generally recognized as granuloma, and formerly described under the names *mycosis fungoides, inflammatory fungoid neoplasm,* and several others. It is characterized usually by symptoms of an eczematous, urticarial, and erysipelatous nature, and by the sudden or gradual appearance of pinkish or reddish, tubercular, nodular, lobulated, or furrowed tumors or flat infiltrations, which may disappear by involution or may be followed by ulceration; several or a larger number of the growths present a mushroom, papillomatous, or fungoid appearance, sometimes roughly resembling the cut part of a tomato. In most cases the tumor stage of the malady is not reached for two or more years; in exceptional instances, however, they appear in the first few months. The lesions, especially in their early stages, are, as a rule, accompanied with more or less burning and itching. [Pg 243]

State the prognosis and treatment of granuloma fungoides.

The malady may last for several years or much longer, a fatal termination, with rare exceptions, sooner or later taking place. After the tumor stage is well established, the patient usually succumbs in from several months to one or two years.

Fig. 65.

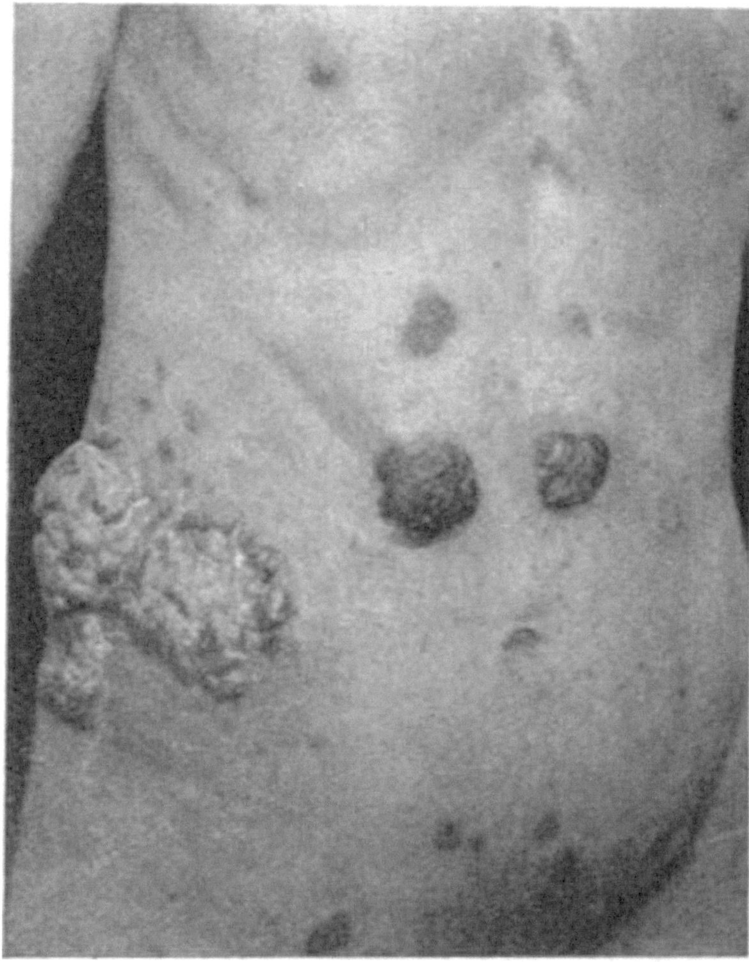

Granuloma Fungoides.

Treatment consists of tonics, if indicated, and the administration of arsenic, preferably hypodermically, and Röntgen-ray exposures, along with the application of mild antiseptics, and operative interference when necessary or advisable. [Pg 244]

CLASS VII.—NEUROSES.

Hyperæsthesia.

What is hyperæsthesia?

By hyperæsthesia is meant increased cutaneous sensibility. It is usually more or less localized, and is met with as a symptom in functional and organic nervous diseases.

Dermatalgia.

(*Synonyms:* Neuralgia of the Skin; Rheumatism of the Skin; Dermalgia.)

What do you understand by dermatalgia?

By dermatalgia is meant a tender or painful condition of the skin unattended by structural change. It is commonly limited to a small area, and is usually symptomatic of functional or organic nervous disease. As an idiopathic affection it is looked upon as of a rheumatic origin.

Treatment depends upon the cause.

Anæsthesia.

What is anæsthesia?

Anæsthesia is a diminution, comparative or complete, of cutaneous sensibility. It is usually localized, and is met with in the course of certain nervous affections. It is also encountered in leprosy, morphœa and like diseases.

Pruritus.

What do you understand by pruritus?

Pruritus is a functional disease of the skin, the sole symptom of which is itching, there being no structural change. [Pg 245]

Describe the symptoms of pruritus.

The sole and essential symptom is itchiness, usually more or less paroxysmal, and worse at night. There are no primary structural lesions, but in severe and persistent cases the parts become so irritated by continued scratching that secondary lesions, such as papules and slight thickening and infiltration, may result. It is much more common in advanced life—*pruritus senilis*. In such cases, as well as in those cases in younger and middle-aged individuals in which the itchiness develops at the approach of cold weather and disappears upon the coming of the warm season (*pruritus hiemalis*), the pruritus is usually more or less generalized, although not infrequently in the latter the legs are specially involved.

In some individuals an attack of pruritus, of variable intensity, lasting from five to thirty minutes, comes on immediately after a bath (*bath-pruritus*). It is usually confined to the legs from the hips down.

Is pruritus always more or less generalized?

No; not infrequently the itching is limited to the genital region (*pruritus scroti, pruritus vulvæ*) or to the anus (*pruritus ani*).

To what may pruritus often be ascribed?

To digestive and intestinal derangements, hepatic disorders, the uric acid diathesis, gestation, diabetes mellitus, and a depraved state of the nervous system.

Pruritus vulvæ is at times due to irritating discharges, and pruritus ani occasionally to hemorrhoids and seat-worms.

Is there any difficulty in the diagnosis of pruritus?

No. The subjective symptom of itching without the presence of structural lesions is diagnostic. In those severe and persistent cases in which excoriations and papules have resulted from the scratching, the history of the case, together with its course, must be considered. Care should be taken not to confound it with pediculosis. In this latter the excoriations usually have a somewhat peculiar distribution, being most abundant on those parts of the body with which the clothing lies closely in contact. (See Pediculosis corporis.) [Pg 246] In pruritus of the genitocrural region the possibility of pediculi being the cause must be kept in mind; an examination of the parts for the parasite or for ova (attached to the hairs) would prevent error. (See Pediculosis pubis.)

What prognosis would you give in pruritus?

In the majority of cases the condition responds to proper treatment, but in others it proves rebellious. The prognosis depends, in fact, upon the removability of the cause. Temporary relief may always be given by external applications.

How would you treat pruritus?

With systemic remedies directed toward a removal or modification of the etiological factors, and, for the temporary relief of the itching, suitable antipruritic applications. In obscure cases, quinia, salophen, lithia salts, calcium chloride, belladonna, nux vomica, arsenic, pilocarpine, and general galvanization may be variously tried. Alkalies prove useful in many cases.

Exceptionally, the relief furnished by external treatment is more or less permanent.

Name the important antipruritic applications.

Alkaline baths; lotions of carbolic acid (ʒj-ʒiij to Oj), of resorcin (ʒj-ʒiv to Oj), of liquor carbonis detergens (℥j-℥iv to Oj), and liquor picis alkalinus (ʒj-ʒiv to Oj), used cautiously. One or several ounces of alcohol and one or two drachms of glycerin in each pint of these lotions will often be of advantage, as the following:—

℞ Ac. carbolici, ... ʒj-ʒiij Gylcerinæ, ... fʒij Alcoholis, ... f℥ij Aquæ, ... q.s. ad. .... Oj. M.

Various dusting-powders, alone or in conjunction with the lotions.

And in some cases, especially those in which the skin is unnaturally dry, ointments may be used, such as equal parts of lard, lanolin, and petrolatum, to the ounce of which may be added from five to thirty grains of carbolic acid, three to twenty grains of thymol, ten to thirty minims of chloroform, or two to ten grains of menthol. [Pg 247]

What external applications are to be used in the local varieties of pruritus?

In *pruritus ani* and *pruritus vulvæ*, in addition to the various applications above, a cocaine ointment, one to ten grains to the ounce, a strong solution of the same (gr. v-xx to ℥j), and an ointment containing ten to thirty minims of the oil of peppermint to the ounce; sponging with hot water, often affords temporary relief.

In pruritus vulvæ, moreover, astringent applications and injections of zinc sulphate, alum, tannic or acetic acid, in the strength commonly employed for vaginal injections, are at times curative.

In bath-pruritus weak glycerine lotions, and an ointment containing a few grains of thymol and menthol to the ounce sometimes give moderate relief. Turkish baths are sometimes free from subsequent pruritus.

CLASS VIII.—PARASITIC AFFECTIONS.

Tinea Favosa.

(*Synonym:* Favus.)

What is tinea favosa?

Tinea favosa, or favus, is a contagious vegetable-parasitic disease of the skin, characterized by pin-head to pea-sized, friable, umbilicated, cup-shaped yellow crusts, each usually perforated by a hair.

Upon what parts and at what age is favus observed?

It is usually met with upon the scalp, but it may occur upon any part of the integument. Occasionally the nails are invaded. It is seen at all ages, but is much more common in children.

Describe the symptoms of favus of the scalp.

The disease begins as a superficial inflammation or hyperæmic spot, more or less circumscribed, slightly scaly, and which is soon followed by the formation of yellowish points about the hair follicles, surrounding the hair shaft. These yellowish points or crusts increase in size, become usually as large as small peas, are cup-shaped, with the convex side pressing down upon the papillary layer, and the [Pg 248] concave side raised several lines above the level of the skin; they are umbilicated, friable, sulphur-colored, and usually each cup or disc is perforated by a hair. Upon removal or detachment, the underlying surface is found to be somewhat excavated, reddened, atrophied and sometimes suppurating. As the disease progresses the crusting becomes more or less confluent, forming irregular masses of thick, yellowish, mortar-like crusts or accumulations, having a peculiar, characteristic odor—that of mice, or stale, damp straw. The hairs are involved early in the disease, become brittle, lustreless, break off and fall out. In some instances, especially near the border of the crusts, are seen pustules or suppurating points. *Atrophy* and more or less actual *scarring* are sooner or later noted.

Itching, variable as to degree, is usually present.

What is the course of favus of the scalp?

Persistent and slowly progressive.

Fig. 66.

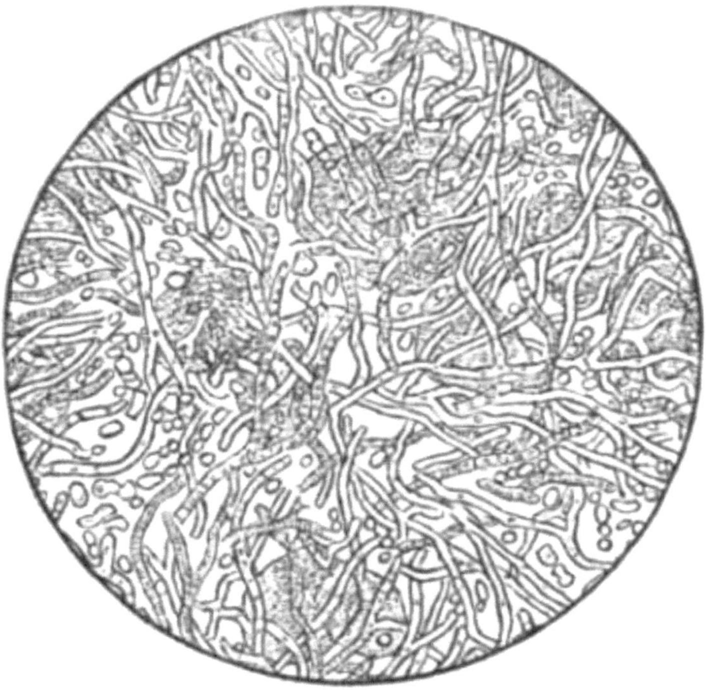

Achorion Schönleinii X 450. (*After Duhring.*)
Showing simple mycelium, in various stages of development, and free spores.

What are the symptoms of favus when seated upon the general surface?

The symptoms are essentially similar to those upon the scalp, modified somewhat by the anatomical differences of the parts. [Pg 249] The *nails*, when affected, become yellowish, more or less thickened, brittle and opaque (*tinea favosa unguium, onychomycosis favosa*).

To what is favus due?

Solely to the invasion of the cutaneous structures, especially the epidermal portion, by the vegetable parasite, the *achorion Schönleinii*.

It is contagious. It is a somewhat rare disease in the native-born, being chiefly observed among the foreign poor. The nails are rarely affected primarily.

It is also met with in the lower animals, from which it is doubtless not infrequently communicated to man.

What are the diagnostic features of favus?

The yellow, and often cup-shaped, crusts, brittleness and loss of hair, atrophy, and the history.

Fig. 67.

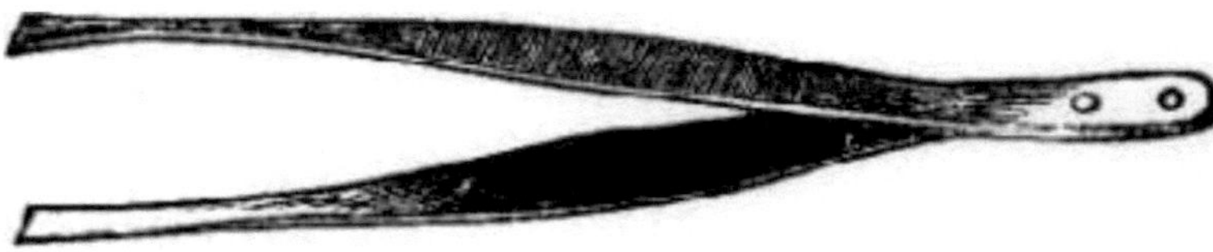

Epilating Forceps.

How would you distinguish favus from eczema and ringworm?

From eczema by the condition of the affected hair, the atrophic and scar-like areas, the odor, and the history. From ringworm by the crusting and the atrophy. In this latter disease there is usually but slight scaliness, and rarely any scarring.

Finally, if necessary, a microscopic examination of the crusts may be made.

State the method of examination for fungus.

A portion of the crust is moistened with liquor potassæ and examined with a power of three to five hundred diameters. The fungus, (achorion Schönleinii), consisting of mycelium and spores, is luxuriant and is readily detected.

State the prognosis of favus..

Upon the scalp, favus is extremely chronic and rebellious to treatment, [Pg 250] and a cure in six to twelve months may be considered satisfactory; in neglected cases permanent baldness, atrophy, and scarring sooner or later result. Although favus of the scalp persists into adult life, it becomes less active and, finally, as a rule, gradually disappears, leaving behind scarred or atrophic bald areas.

Upon the general surface it usually responds readily to treatment, excepting favus of the nails, which is always obstinate.

How is favus of the scalp treated?

Treatment is entirely local and consists in keeping the parts free from crusts, in epilation and applications of a parasiticide.

The crusts are removed by oily applications and soap-and-water washings. The hair on and around the diseased parts is to be kept closely cut, and, when practicable, depilation, or extraction of the affected hairs, is advised; this latter is, in most cases, essential to a cure. Remedial applications—the so-called parasiticides—are, as a rule, to be made twice daily. If an ointment is used, it is to be thoroughly rubbed in; if a lotion, it is to be dabbed on for several minutes and allowed to soak in.

Name the most important parasiticides.

Corrosive sublimate, one to four grains to an ounce of alcohol and water; carbolic acid, one part to three or more parts of glycerine; a ten per cent. oleate of mercury; ointments of ammoniated mercury, sulphur and tar; and sulphurous acid, pure or diluted. The following is valuable:—

> ℞ Sulphur, præcip., ... ʒij Saponis viridis, Ol.
> cadini, ...āā................ ʒj Adipis,
> .... ℥ss. M.

Chrysarobin is a valuable remedy, but must be used with caution; it may be employed as an ointment, five to ten per cent. strength, as a rubber plaster, or as a paint, a drachm to an ounce of gutta-percha solution. Formalin, weakened or full strength, has been extolled. Some observers have experimentally tried the effect of *x*-ray exposure with alleged good results, pushing the treatment to the point of producing depilation; if used great caution should be exercised. [Pg 251]

How is favus upon the general surface to be treated?

In the same general manner as favus of the scalp, but the remedies employed should be somewhat weaker. In favus of the nail frequent and close paring of the affected part and the application, twice daily, of one of the milder parasiticides, will eventually lead to a good result.

Is constitutional treatment of any value in favus?

It is questionable, but in debilitated subjects tonics, especially cod-liver oil, may be prescribed with the hope of aiding the external applications.

Tinea Trichophytina.

(*Synonym:* Ringworm.)

What is tinea trichophytina?

Tinea trichophytina, or ringworm, is a contagious, vegetable-parasitic disease due to the invasion of the cutaneous structures by the vegetable parasite, the trichophyton, or the microsporon Audouinii.

Do the clinical characters of ringworm vary according to the part affected?

Yes, often considerably; thus upon the scalp, upon the general surface, and upon the bearded region, the disease usually presents totally different appearances.

Describe the symptoms of ringworm as it occurs upon non-hairy portions of the body.

Ringworm of the general surface (*tinea trichophytina corporis, tinea circinata*) appears as one or more small, slightly-elevated, sharply-limited, somewhat scaly, hyperæmic spots, with, rarely, minute papules, vesico-papules, or vesicles, especially at the circumference. The patch spreads in a uniform manner peripherally, is slightly scaly, and tends to clear in the centre, assuming a ring-like appearance. When coming under observation, the patches are usually from one-half to one inch in diameter, the central portion pale or pale red, and the outer portion more or less elevated, hyperæmic and somewhat scaly. As commonly noted one, several or more patches are present. After reaching a certain size they may [Pg 252] remain stationary, or in exceptional cases may tend to spontaneous disappearance. At times when close together, several may merge and form a large, irregular, gyrate patch.

Itching, usually slight, may or may not be present.

Exceptionally ringworm appears as a markedly inflammatory pustular circumscribed patch, formerly thought to be a distinct affection and described under the name of *conglomerate pustular folliculitis*. It consists of a flat carbuncular or kerion-like inflammation, somewhat elevated, and usually a dime to silver dollar in area. The most common seats are the back of the hands and the buttocks. The surface is cribriform, and a purulent secretion may be pressed out from follicular openings.

Fig. 68.

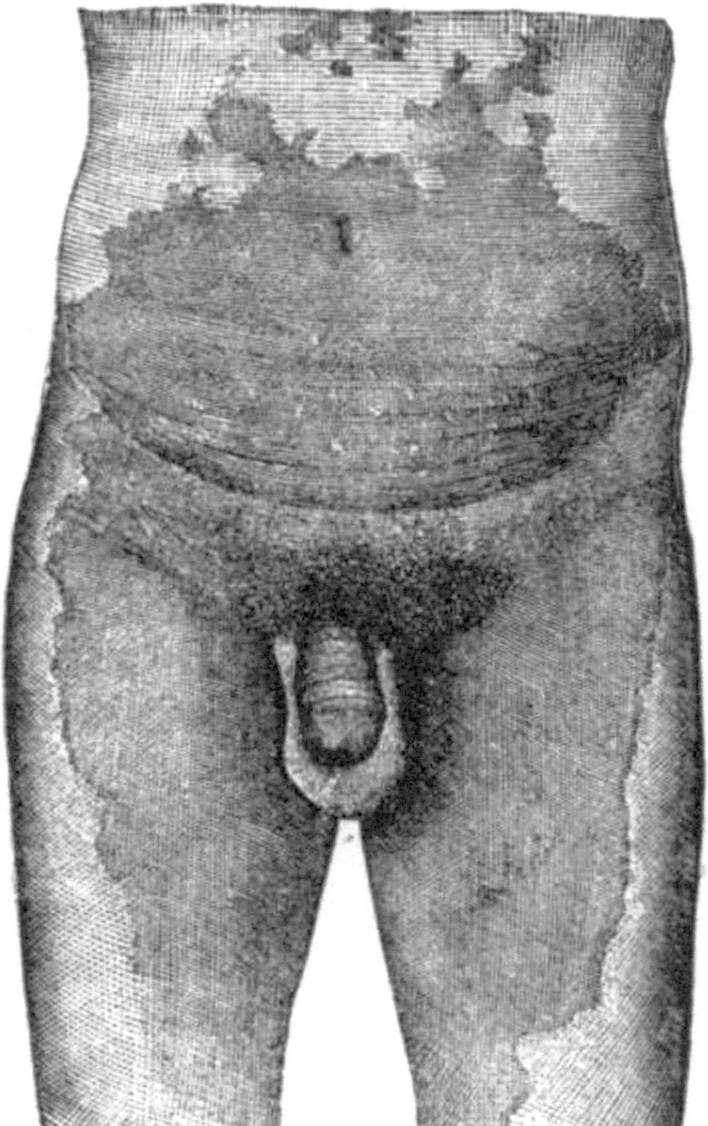

Tinea trichophytina cruris—so-called eczema marginatum—of unusually extensive development. (*After Piffard.*)

Describe the symptoms of ringworm when occurring about the thighs and scrotum.

In adults, more especially males, the inner portion of the upper part of the thighs and scrotum (*tinea trichophytina cruris,* so-called [Pg 253] *eczema marginatum*) may be attacked, and here the affection, favored by heat and moisture, develops rapidly and may soon lose its ordinary clinical appearances, the inflammatory symptoms becoming especially prominent. The whole of this region may become involved, presenting all the symptoms of a true eczema; the border, however, is sharply defined, and usually one or more outlying patches of the ordinary clinical type of the disease may be seen.

Describe the symptoms of ringworm when involving the nails.

In ringworm of the nails (*tinea trichophytina unguium*) these structures become soft or brittle, yellowish, opaque and thickened the changes taking place mainly about the free borders. Ringworm on other parts usually coexists.

Describe the symptoms of ringworm as it occurs upon the scalp.

Ringworm of the scalp (*tinea trichophytina capitis, tinea tonsurans*) begins usually in the same manner as that upon the general surface, but, as a rule, much more insidiously. Sooner or later, however, the hair and follicles are invaded by the fungus, and in consequence the hair falls out or becomes brittle and breaks off. The follicles, except in long-standing cases, are slightly elevated and prominent, and the patch may have a puffed or goose-flesh appearance. In addition, there is slight scaliness.

Describe the appearances of a typical patch of ringworm of the scalp.

The patch is rounded, grayish, somewhat scaly, and slightly elevated; the follicles are somewhat prominent; there is more or less alopecia, with here and there broken, gnawed-off-looking hairs, some of which may be broken off just at the outlet of the follicles and more or less surrounded by a whitish or grayish-white dust. This type is produced by the small-spore fungus—microsporon.

Does ringworm of the scalp always present typical appearances?

Not invariably. In some cases the patch or patches may become [Pg 254] almost completely bald, and in others a tendency to the formation of pustules, with more or less crust-formation, may be seen. The affection may also appear as small scattered spots or points.

Fig. 69.

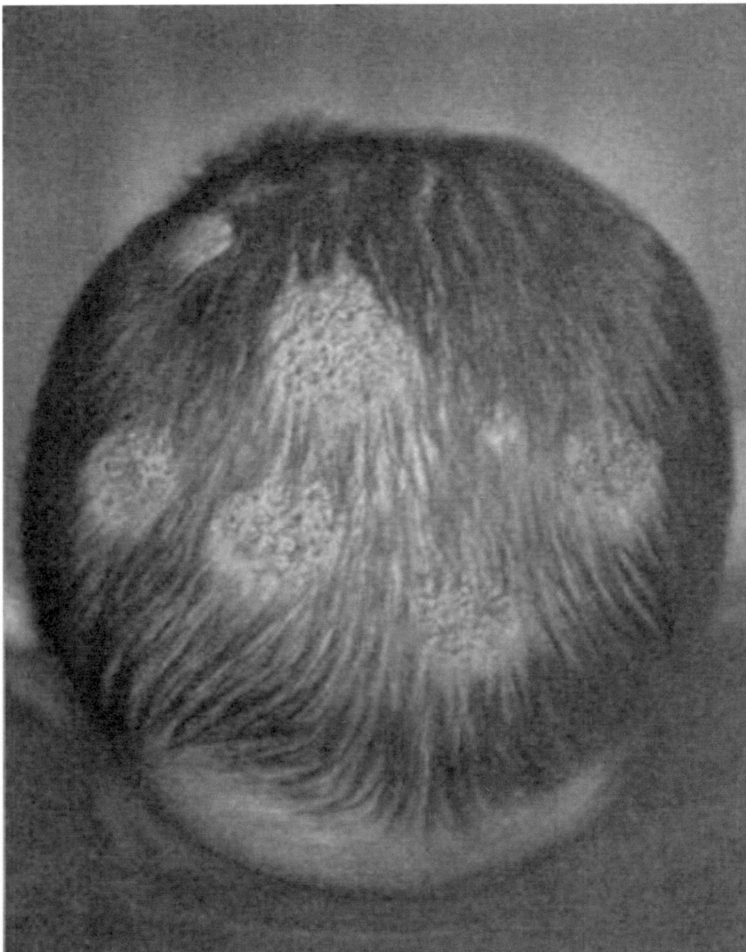

Ringworm (rather inflammatory type, and produced by the trichophyton).

[Pg 255] The markedly inflammatory and pustular types are produced by the large-spore fungus—trichophyton.

What is tinea kerion?

Tinea kerion (*kerion*) is a markedly inflammatory type of ringworm of the scalp involving the deeper tissues, appearing as a more or less bald, rounded, inflammatory, œdematous, boggy, honeycombed tumor, discharging from the follicular openings a mucoid secretion.

Does ringworm of the scalp ever occur in adults?

No. (Extremely rare exceptions.)

Fig. 70.

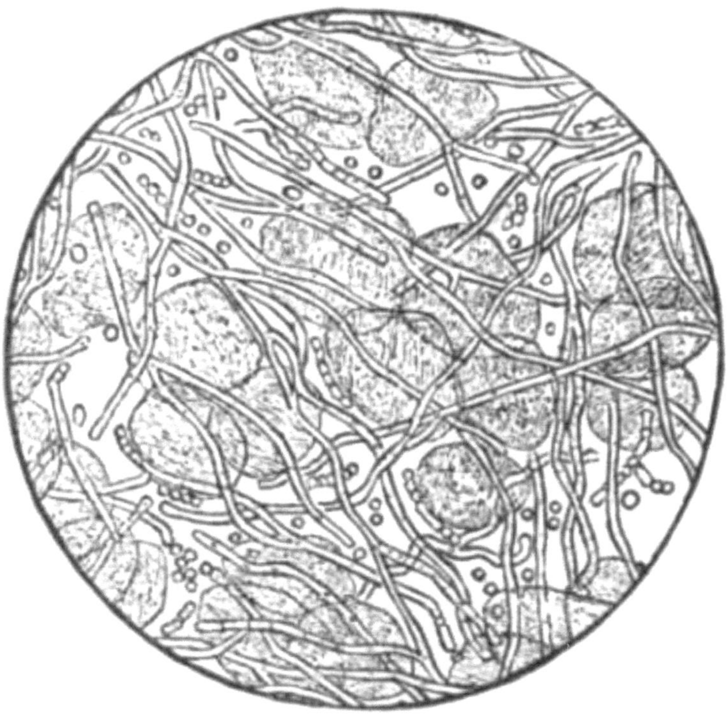

Ringworm Fungus (Trichophyton) x 450. (*After Duhring.*)
As found in epidermic scrapings of ringworm, showing mycelium and spores.

Describe the symptoms of ringworm of the bearded region.

Ringworm of the bearded region (*tinea trichophytina barbæ, tinea sycosis, parasitic sycosis, barber's itch*) begins usually in the same manner as ringworm on other parts, as one or more rounded, slightly scaly, hyperæmic patches. In rare instances the disease may persist as such, with very little tendency to involve the hairs and follicles; but, as a rule, the hairy structures are soon invaded, many of the hairs breaking off, and many falling out. From involvement of the [Pg 256] follicles, more or less subcutaneous swelling ensues, the parts assuming a distinctly *lumpy and nodular* condition. The skin is usually considerably reddened, often having a glossy appearance, and studded with few or numerous pustules. The nodules tend, ordinarily, to break down and discharge, at one or more of the follicular openings, a glairy, glutinous, purulent material, which may dry to thick, adherent crusts.

Fig. 71.

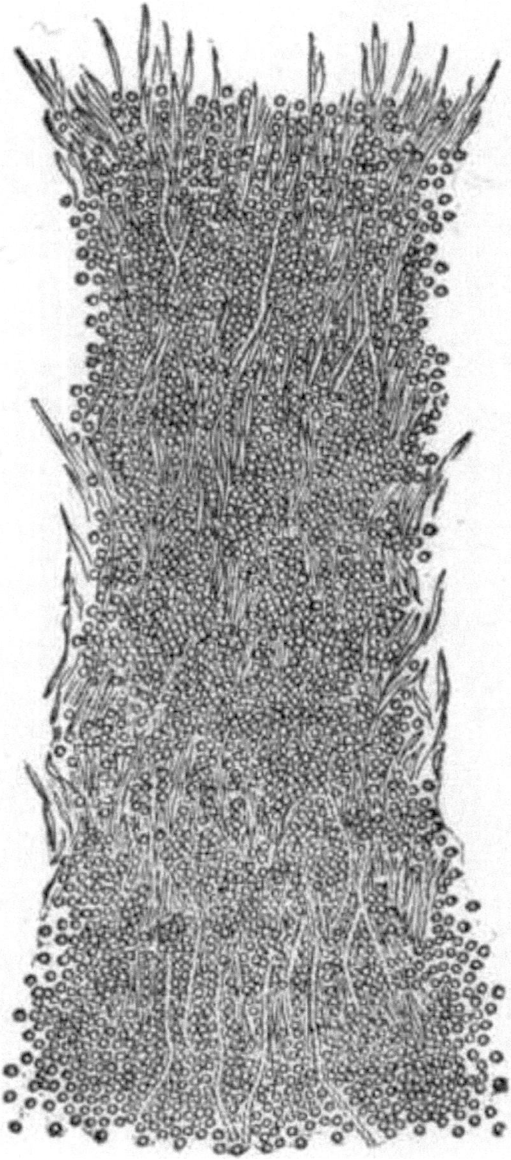

Ringworm Fungus (Microsporon) x 500. (*After Duhring.*)
Short, broken-off hair of scalp invaded with masses of free spores.

[Pg 257] The disease may be limited to one patch, or a large area, even to the extent of the whole bearded region, becomes involved. The upper lip is rarely invaded. Ringworm of the bearded region is due to the trichophyton.

Fig. 72.

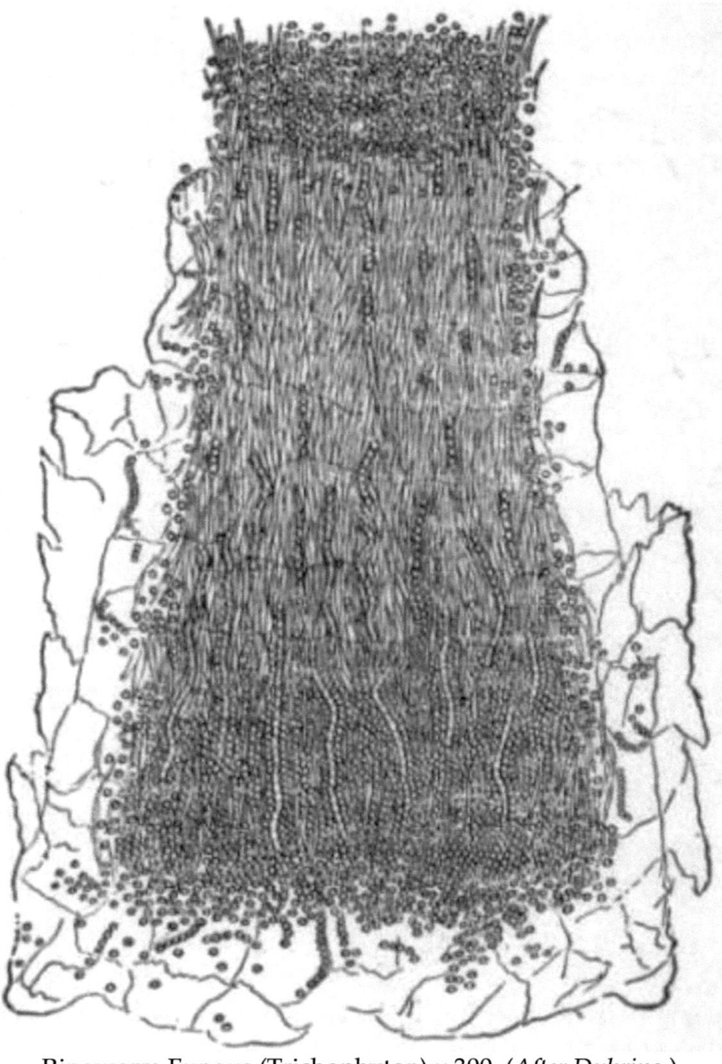

Ringworm Fungus (Trichophyton) x 300. (*After Duhring.*)
Short, stout hair of beard, with the root-sheath attached, showing free spores and chains of spores.

To what is ringworm due?

To the presence and growth in the cutaneous structures of a vegetable parasite. Although the disease is contagious, individuals differ considerably as to susceptibility. It is much more common in [Pg 258] children than in those past the age of puberty, ringworm of the scalp being limited to the former (rare exceptions), and tinea sycosis being a disease of the male adult.

Until recently the ringworm was thought to be due to but one fungus—the trichophyton; it is now known that there are several forms of fungi, the main forms being the small-spored (microsporon Audouini) and the large-spored (trichophyton). Of this latter there are two main subvarieties—endothrix and ectothrix. The small-spored fungus is found as the cause in the majority of scalp cases; the endothrix also commonly invades the scalp integument. The ectothrix variety is usually derived directly or indirectly from domestic animals, and is chiefly responsible for body-ringworm, and for suppurative ringworm, whether upon the bearded region or elsewhere.

What is the pathology of ringworm?

On the general surface the fungus has its seat in the epidermis, especially in the corneous layer; upon the scalp and bearded region the epidermis, hair-shaft, root and follicle are invaded. The inflammatory action may vary considerably in different cases, and at different times in the same case.

The fungus consists of mycelium and spores. In the epidermic scrapings it is never to be found in abundance, and the mycelium predominates, while in affected hairs the spores and chains of spores are almost exclusively seen, and are usually present in great profusion.

How do you examine for the fungus?

The scrapings or hair should be moistened with liquor potassæ, and examined with a power from three hundred diameters upward.

How is ringworm of the general surface to be distinguished from eczema, psoriasis and seborrhœa?

By the growth and characters of the patch, the slight scaliness, the tendency to disappear in the centre, by the history, and, if necessary, by a microscopic examination of the scales.

How is ringworm of the scalp to be distinguished from alopecia areata, favus, eczema, seborrhœa, and psoriasis?

By the peculiar clinical features of ringworm on this region—the [Pg 259] slight scaliness, broken hair and hair stumps, with a certain amount of baldness—and in doubtful cases by a microscopical examination of the hairs.

In favus, although the same condition of the hair is noted, the yellow, cup-shaped crusts, and the presence of the atrophic areas in that disease are pathognomonic.

How is ringworm of the bearded region to be distinguished from eczema and sycosis?

By the peculiar lumpiness of the parts, the brittleness of the hair, more or less hair loss, and the history.

The superficial type of ringworm sycosis—those cases in which the disease remains a surface disease—is readily distinguished, as the symptoms are essentially the same as ringworm of non-hairy parts, except that some of the hairs in the areas may become invaded and break off or fall out.

In doubtful cases recourse may be had to microscopical examination.

What is the prognosis of ringworm of these several parts?

When upon the general surface, the disease usually responds rapidly to therapeutical applications; upon the scalp it is always a stubborn affection, and, as a rule, requires several months to a year of energetic treatment to effect a cure. In this latter region the disease will disappear spontaneously as the age of fifteen or sixteen is reached. Tinea sycosis yields in most instances in the course of several weeks or a few months.

Is ringworm of these several parts treated with the same remedies?

As a rule, yes; but the strength must be modified. The scalp will stand strong applications, as will likewise the bearded region; upon non-hairy portions the remedies should be used somewhat weaker. They should be applied twice daily; ointments, if used, being well rubbed in, and lotions thoroughly dabbed on.

How would you treat ringworm of the general surface?

By applications of the milder parasiticides, such as a ten to fifteen per cent. solution of sodium hyposulphite; carbolic acid, five to thirty grains to the ounce of water, or lard; a saturated solution of [Pg 260] boric acid; ointments of tar, sulphur and mercury, official strength or weakened with lard; and tincture of iodine, pure or diluted.

When occurring upon the upper and inner part of the thighs (so-called eczema marginatum), the same remedies are to be employed, but usually stronger. Deserving of special mention is a lotion of corrosive sublimate, one to four grains to the ounce; or the same remedy, in the same proportion, may be used in tincture of myrrh or benzoin, and painted on the parts.

How would you treat ringworm of the scalp?

By occasional soap-and-hot-water washing; by extraction of the involved hairs, when practicable; by carbolic acid or boric acid lotions to the whole scalp, so as to limit, as much as possible, the spread of the disease; and by daily (or twice daily) applications to the patches and involved areas of a parasiticide. The following are the most valuable: the oleate of mercury, with lard or lanolin, in varying strength, from ten to twenty per cent.; carbolic acid, with one to three or more parts of glycerine or oil; corrosive sublimate, in solution in alcohol and water, one to four grains to the ounce; sulphur ointment; and citrine ointment, with one or two parts of lard. Chrysarobin is a valuable remedy, but is to be employed with care; it may be prescribed as a rubber plaster, or in a solution of gutta-percha, or as an ointment, ten to fifteen per cent. strength. β-naphthol in ointment form, five to fifteen per cent. strength, is also useful. An excellent application for beginning areas on the scalp is a solution of the red iodide of mercury in iodine tincture, one to three grains to an ounce.

A compound ointment, containing several of the active remedies named, is convenient for dispensary practice, such as:—

℞ β-naphthol, ... ʒss-ʒj Ol. cadini, ... ʒj Ungt. sulphuris, ... q.s. ad. ℥j. M.

In that form known as tinea kerion mild applications are demanded at first; later the same treatment as in the ordinary type.

How is ringworm of the bearded region to be treated?

On the same general plan and with the same remedies (excepting [Pg 261] chrysarobin) as in ringworm of the scalp. Depilation is to be practised as an essential part of the treatment. Special mention may be made of an ointment of oleate of mercury, sulphur ointment, a lotion of sodium hyposulphite (ʒj-℥j), and a lotion of corrosive sublimate (gr. j-iv to ℥j). The *x*-ray has been used in ringworm of this region with alleged success, pushing it to the production of a mild erythema and depilation. The above methods are, however, usually successful, and are without risk of damage.

How is the certainty of an apparent cure in ringworm of the scalp or bearded region to be determined?

By the continued absence of roughness and of broken hairs and stumps, and by microscopical examination of the new-growing hairs from time to time for several weeks after discontinuance of treatment.

Cure of ringworm of the general surface is usually self-evident.

Is systemic treatment of aid in the cure of ringworm?

It is doubtful, although in children in a depraved state of health the disease is often noted to be especially stubborn, and in such cod-liver oil and similar remedies may at times prove of benefit.

Tinea Imbricata.

(*Synonym:* Tokelau Ringworm.)

What is tinea imbricata?

A vegetable parasitic disease of moist tropical countries, characterized by the formation of patches composed of concentrically arranged, imbricated, scaly rings. It may begin at one or several points as a brownish, slightly raised spot, spreading peripherally; the renewed epidermis of the central part of the patch goes again through the same process; the result is a small or large area of concentrically arranged, imbricated, slightly scaly eruption. Several such areas fusing together may cover a large part of the surface, the ring-like arrangement being sometimes more or less completely lost. The malady is chronic. There may be a variable degree of itching. The cause of the disease, which is of a contagious nature, is a [Pg 262] vegetable parasite closely similar to the trichophyton. The treatment is by the parasiticides, being essentially the same, in fact, as ringworm.

Tinea Versicolor.

(*Synonyms:* Pityriasis Versicolor; Chromophytosis.)

What is tinea versicolor?

Tinea versicolor is a vegetable-parasitic disease of the skin, characterized by variously-sized and shaped, slightly scaly, macular patches of a yellowish-fawn color, and occurring for the most part upon the upper portion of the trunk.

Describe the symptoms of tinea versicolor.

The disease begins as one or more yellowish macular points; these, in the course of weeks or months, gradually extend, and, together with other patches that arise, may form a more or less continuous sheet of eruption. There is slight scaliness, always insignificant and furfuraceous in character, and at times, except upon close inspection, scarcely perceptible. The color of the patches is pale or brownish-yellow; in rare instances, in those of delicate skin, there may be more or less hyperæmia, and in consequence the eruption is of a reddish tinge. The number of patches varies; there may be but a few, or, on the other hand, a profusion. Slight itching, especially when the parts are warm, is usually present.

Does the eruption of tinea versicolor show predilection for any special region?

Yes; the upper part of the trunk, especially anteriorly, is the usual seat of the eruption, but in exceptional instances the neck, axillæ, the arms, the whole trunk, the genitocrural region and poplitea, and in rare cases even the lower part of the face, may become invaded.

What course does tinea versicolor pursue?

Persistent, but somewhat variable; as a rule, however, slowly progressive and lasting for years.

To what is tinea versicolor due?

To a vegetable fungus—the *microsporon furfur*. [Pg 263] The affection is tolerably common, and occurs in all parts of the world. With rare exceptions, it is a disease of adults, and while looked upon as contagious, must be so to an extremely slight degree.

Fig. 73.

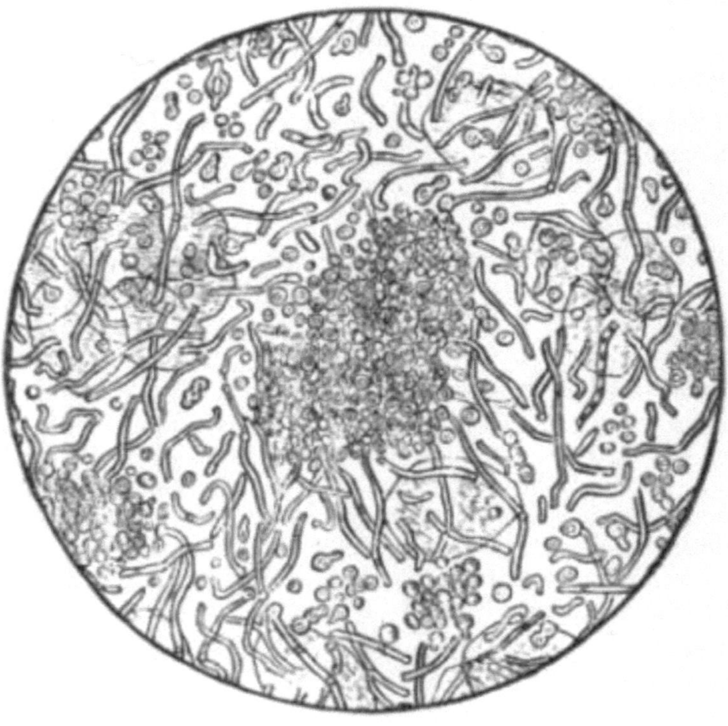

Microsporon Furfur x 400. (*After Duhring.*)
Showing mycelium in various stages of development, groups of spores and free spores.

What is the pathology?

The fungus, consisting of mycelium and spores, the latter showing a marked tendency to aggregate, invades the superficial portion of the epidermis.

Is tinea versicolor readily diagnosticated?

Yes; if the color, peculiar characters and distribution of the eruption are kept in mind.

It is not to be confounded with vitiligo, chloasma, or the macular syphiloderm. If in doubt, have recourse to the microscope.

State the method of examination for fungus.

The scrapings are taken from a patch, moistened with liquor potassæ, and examined with a power of three to five hundred diameters.

State the prognosis of tinea versicolor.

With proper management the disease is readily curable. Relapses are not uncommon. [Pg 264]

Fig. 74.

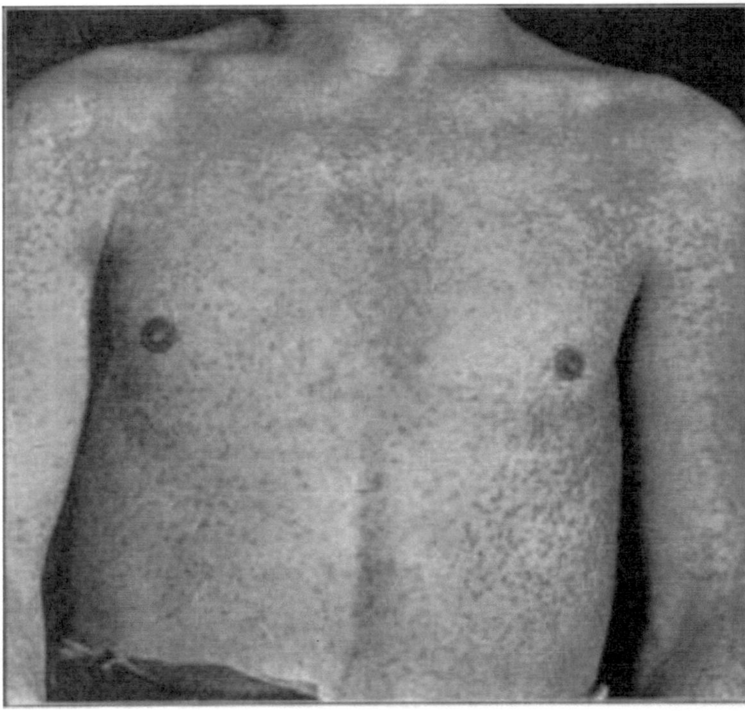

Tinea versicolor.

What is the treatment of tinea versicolor?

It consists in daily washing with soap and hot water (and in obstinate cases with sapo viridis instead of the ordinary soap) and application of a lotion of—sulphite or hyposulphite of sodium, a drachm to the ounce; sulphurous acid, pure or diluted; carbolic acid, or resorcin, ten to twenty grains to the ounce of water and alcohol; or corrosive sublimate, one to three grains to the ounce of water. Sulphur and ammoniated-mercury ointments are also serviceable. The following used alone, simply as a soap, or in conjunction with a lotion, is often of special value:—

℞ Sulphur, præcip., ... ʒiv Saponis viridis, ... ʒxii. M.

[Pg 265] After the disease is apparently cured, an occasional remedial application should be made for several months, in order to guard against the possibility of a relapse.

Erythrasma.

Erythrasma.

Describe erythrasma.

Erythrasma is an extremely rare disease, due to the presence and growth in the epidermic structures of the vegetable parasite—the *microsporon minutissimum*. It is characterized by small and large, slightly furfuraceous, reddish-yellow or reddish-brown patches, occurring usually on warm and moist parts, such as the axillary, inguinal, anal and genitocrural regions. It is slowly progressive and persistent, but is without disturbing symptoms other than occasional slight itching.

Fig. 75.

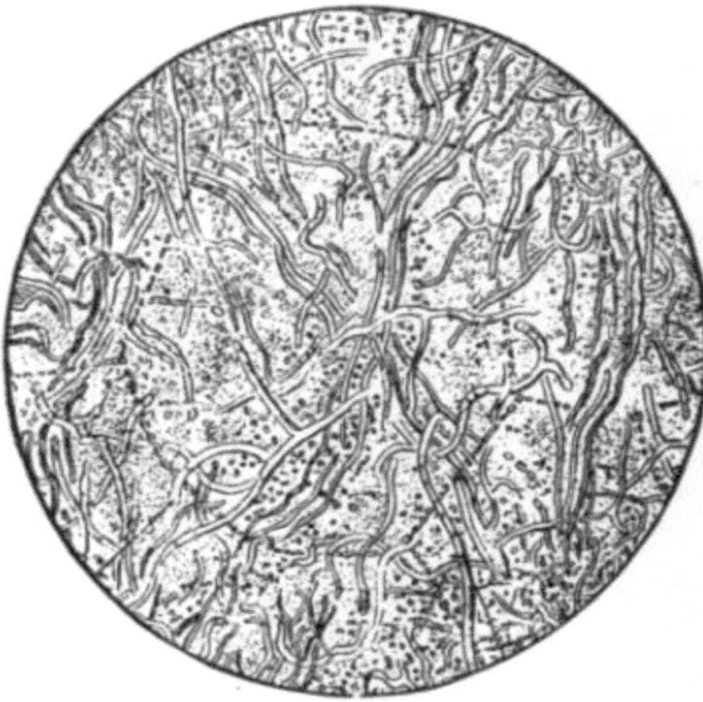

Microsporon Minutissimum x 1000. (*After Riehl.*)

Treatment, which is rapidly effective, is the same as that employed in tinea versicolor.

Dhobie Itch.

Dhobie itch is a name used in certain tropical countries to designate a somewhat peculiar itching eruption of the genitocrural and axillary regions, and by some also a similar eruption about the feet. [Pg 266] It consists of a dermatitis of variable degree, usually with a festooned, irregular border, with considerable itching. It is believed that such cases are variously due to the trichophyton of ringworm, to the microsporon furfur of tinea versicolor, to the microsporon minutissimus of erythrasma, and to other parasites.

Actinomycosis.

Describe actinomycosis.

Actinomycosis of the skin is an affection due to the ray fungus, and characterized by a sluggish, red, nodular, or lumpy infiltration, usually with a tendency to break down and form sinuses. The affection may involve almost any part, but its most common site is about the jaw, neck, and face. As a rule, the first evidence is a hard subcutaneous swelling or infiltration, which may increase slightly or considerably. The overlying skin gradually becomes of a sluggish or dark-red color. Softening ensues, and the diseased area breaks down at one or more points, from which there oozes a discharge of a sero-purulent, purulent, or sanguinolent character. In this discharge can be usually noted minute, friable, yellowish or yellowish-gray bodies representing conglomerate collections of the causative fungus.

The course of the malady is commonly slow and insidious. Unless systemic pyemic infection occurs or the fungus elements find their way to the deeper organs or structures the general health remains apparently undisturbed.

What is the treatment?

The administration of moderate to large doses of potassium iodide, conjointly with curetting or excision of the diseased mass. Local applications of iodine solution can also be tried.

Blastomycetic Dermatitis.

What do you understand by blastomycetic dermatitis?

Blastomycetic dermatitis is a rare disease beginning usually as a small papule or nodule, enlarging slowly, breaking down and developing into a verrucous or papillomatous-looking area, similar in appearance

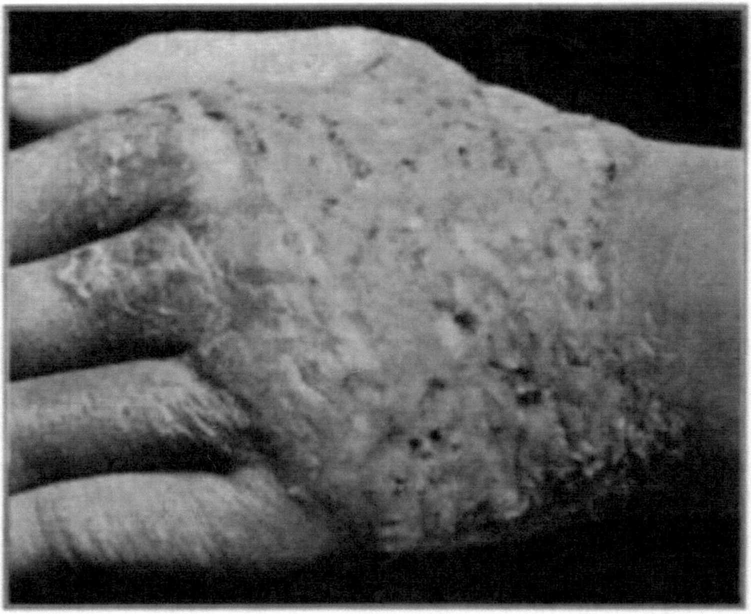

Blastomycetic dermatitis.

[Pg 267] to tuberculosis cutis verrucosa. A muco-purulent or purulent secretion can visually be pressed out from between the papillomatous elevations. It may also present the appearance of a serpiginous lupus vulgaris or syphiloderm. As a rule it is slow in its course. Furuncular or abscess-like formations may develop, usually from secondary infection. The disease is due to the invasion of the cutaneous tissues by the blastomyces.

Treatment consists in administration of moderate to large doses of potassium iodide, and in the employment of antiseptic and parasiticide applications; usually, however, radical treatment, such as employed in lupus vulgaris, may be necessary.

Scabies.

(*Synonym:* The Itch.)

What is scabies?

Scabies, or itch, is a contagious animal-parasitic disease characterized by a multiform eruption of a somewhat peculiar distribution, attended by intense itching.

Describe the symptoms of scabies.

The penetration and presence of the parasites within the cutaneous structures besides often giving rise to several or more complete or imperfectly formed *burrows*, excite varying degrees of irritation, and in consequence the formation of vesicles, papules and pustules, accompanied with more or less intense itching. Secondarily, crusting, and at times a mild or severe grade of dermatitis, may be brought about. The parasite seeks preferably tender and protected situations, as between the fingers, on the wrists, especially the flexor surface, in the folds of the axilla, on the abdomen, about the anal fissure, about the genitalia, and in females also about the nipples, and hence the eruption is most abundant about these regions. The inside of the thighs and the feet are also attacked, as, indeed, may be almost every portion of the body. The scalp and face are not involved; exceptionally, however, these parts are invaded in infants and young children. [Pg 268]

Is the grade of cutaneous irritation the same in all cases of scabies?

No; in those of great cutaneous irritability, especially in children, the skin being more tender, the type of the eruption is usually much more inflammatory. In those predisposed a true eczema may arise, and then, in addition to the characteristic lesions of scabies, eczematous symptoms are superadded; in long-persistent cases, indeed, the burrows and other consequent lesions may be more or less completely masked by the eczematous inflammation, and the true nature of the disease be greatly obscured.

What do you mean by burrows?

Burrows, or *cuniculi*, are tortuous, straight or zigzag, dotted, slightly elevated, dark-gray or blackish thread-like linear formations, varying in length from an eighth to a half an inch.

Fig. 76.

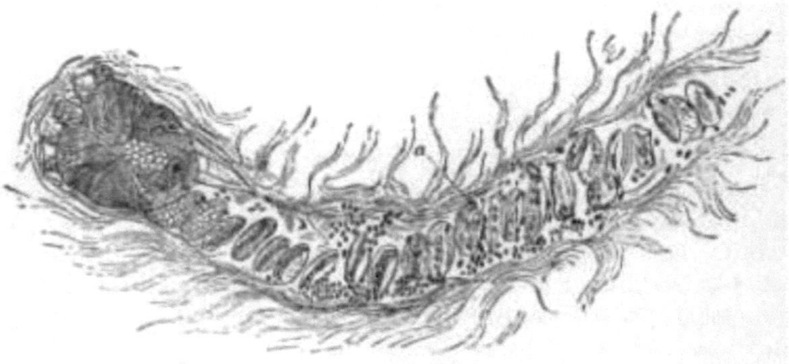

Burrow, or cuniculus, greatly magnified. (*After Kaposi.*)

Showing the mite, ova, empty shells and excrement.

How is a burrow formed?

By the impregnated female parasite, which penetrates the epidermis obliquely to the rete, depositing as it goes along ten or fifteen ova, forming a minute passage or burrow.

Upon what parts are burrows most commonly to be found?

In the interdigital spaces, on the flexor surface of the wrists, about the mammæ in the female, and on the shaft of the penis in the male. [Pg 269]

Are burrows usually present in numbers?

No. Several may be found in a single case, but they are rarely numerous, as the irritation caused by the penetration of the parasites leads either to violent scratching and their destruction, or gives rise to the formation of vesicles and pustules, and consequently their formation is prevented.

What course does scabies pursue?

Chronic and progressive, showing no tendency to spontaneous disappearance.

To what is scabies due?

To the invasion of the cutaneous structures by an animal parasite, the sarcoptes scabiei (*acarus scabiei*). The male mite is never found in the skin and apparently takes no direct part in the production of the symptoms.

Fig. 77. FIG. 78.

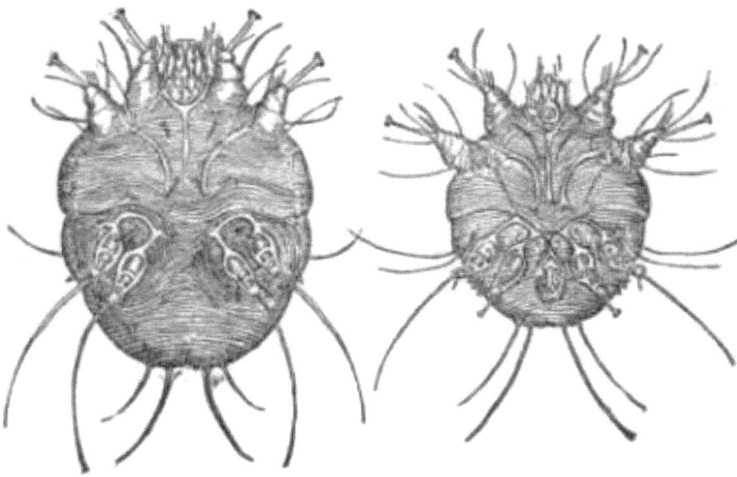

Sarcoptes scabiei x 100. (*After Duhring.*)

Female. Ventral surface. Male.

The disease is contagious to a marked degree, and is most commonly contracted by sleeping with those affected, or by occupying a bed in which an affected person has slept. It occurs, for obvious reasons, usually among the poor, although it is now quite frequently met with among the better classes. [Pg 270]

State the diagnostic features of scabies.

The burrows, the peculiar distribution and the multiformity of the eruption, the progressive development, and usually a history of contagion.

How do vesicular and pustular eczema differ from scabies?

Eczema is usually limited in extent, or irregularly distributed, is distinctly patchy, with often the formation of large diffused areas; it is variable in its clinical behavior, better and worse from time to time, and differs, moreover, in the absence of burrows and of a history of contagion.

How does pediculosis corporis differ from scabies?

In the distribution of the eruption. The pediculi live in the clothing and go to the skin solely for nourishment, and hence the eruption in that condition is upon covered parts, especially those parts with which the clothing lies closely in contact, as around the neck, across the upper part of the back, about the waist and down the outside of the thighs; *the hands are free.*

State the prognosis of scabies.

It is favorable. The disease is readily cured, and, as soon as the parasites and their ova are destroyed, the itching and the secondary symptoms, as a rule, rapidly disappear.

How is scabies treated?

Treatment is entirely external, and consists of a preliminary soap-and-hot-water bath, an application, twice daily for three days, of a remedy destructive to the parasites and ova, and finally another bath.

Inquiry as to others of the family should be made, and, if affected, treated at the same time. The wearing apparel should be looked after—boiled, baked, or sulphur-fumigated.

What remedial applications are employed in scabies?

Sulphur, balsam of Peru, styrax, and β-naphthol, singly or severally combined. In children, or in those of sensitive skin, the following:—

℞ Sulphur. præcip., ... ʒiv Balsam. Peruv., ... ʒij Adipis, Petrolati, ...āā................ ℥iss. M.

[Pg 271] And in adults, or those of non-irritable skin:—

℞ Sulphur, præcip., ... ℥j Balsam. Peruv., ... ℥ss β-Naphthol, ... ʒij Adipis, Petrolati, ...āā......... q.s. ad. .... ℥iv. M.

Styrax is a remedy of value and is commonly employed as an ointment in the strength of one part to two or three parts of lard.

Is one such course of treatment sufficient to bring about a cure?

Yes, in ordinary cases, if the applications have been carefully and thoroughly made; exceptionally, however, some parasites and ova escape destruction, and consequently itching will again begin to show itself at the end of a week or ten days, and a repetition of the treatment become necessary.

Does the secondary dermatitis which is always present in severe cases require treatment?

Only when it is unusually persistent or severe; in such cases the various soothing applications, lotions or ointments employed in acute eczema are to be prescribed.

Is a dermatitis due to too active and prolonged treatment ever mistaken for persistence of the scabies?

Yes.

Pediculosis.

(*Synonyms:* Phtheiriasis; Lousiness.)

Define pediculosis.

Pediculosis is a term applied to that condition of local or general cutaneous irritation due to the presence of the animal parasite, the pediculus, or louse.

Name the several varieties met with.

Three varieties are presented, named according to the parts involved, [Pg 272] pediculosis capitis, pediculosis corporis, and pediculosis pubis; the parasite in each being a distinct species of pediculus.

Pediculosis Capitis.

Describe the symptoms of pediculosis capitis.

Pediculosis capitis (*pediculosis capillitii*), due to the presence of the pediculus capitis, occurs much more frequently in children than in adults. It is characterized by marked itching, and the formation of various inflammatory lesions, such as papules, pustules and excoriations— resulting from the irritation produced by the parasites and from the scratching to which the intense pruritus gives rise. In fact, an eczematous eruption of the pustular type soon results, attended with more or less crust formation. In consequence of the cutaneous irritation the neighboring lymphatic glands may become inflamed and swollen, and in rare cases suppurate. The occipital region is the part which is usually most profusely infested, more especially in young girls and women. In those of delicate skin, especially in children, scattered papules, vesico-papules, pustules, and excoriations may often be seen upon the forehead and neck. In some instances, however, especially in boys, there may be many pediculi present, with but little cutaneous disturbance, the itching being the sole symptom.

Fig. 79.

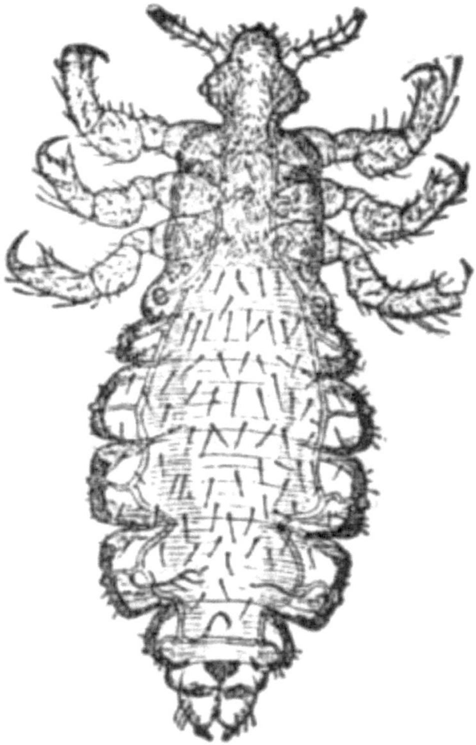

Pediculus Capitis x 25. (*After Duhring.*)

Female. Dorsal surface.

Fig. 80.

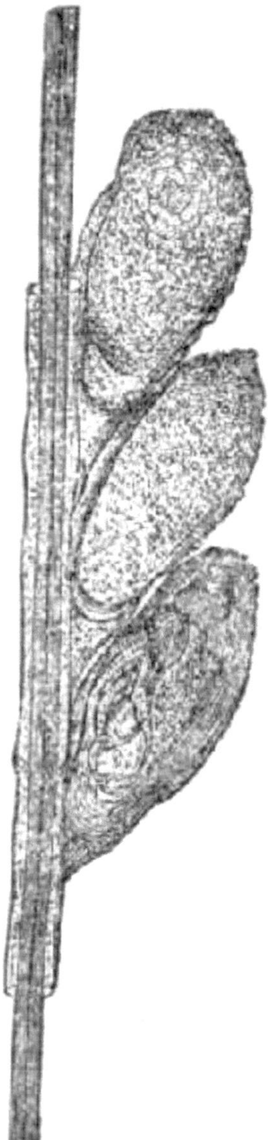

Ova of the headlouse attached to a hair. Magnified. *(After Kaposi.)*

[Pg 273] In addition to the pediculi, which, as a rule, may be readily found, their *ova,* or *nits,* are always to be seen upon the shaft of the hairs, quite firmly attached.

Describe the appearance of the ova.

They are dirty-white or grayish looking, minute, pear-shaped bodies, visible to the naked eye, and fastened upon the shaft of the hairs with the small end toward the root.

Is there any difficulty in the diagnosis of pediculosis capitis?

No. The diagnosis is readily made, as the pediculi are usually to be found without difficulty, and even when they exist in small numbers and are not readily discovered, *the presence of the ova* will indicate the nature of the affection.

Pustular eruptions upon the scalp, especially posteriorly, should always arouse a suspicion of pediculosis. The possibility of the pediculosis being secondary to eczema must not be forgotten.

What is the treatment of pediculosis capitis?

Treatment consists in the application of some remedy destructive to the pediculi and their ova. Crude petroleum is effective, one or two thorough applications over night being usually sufficient; in order to lessen its inflammability, and also to mask its somewhat disagreeable odor, it may be mixed with an equal part of olive oil and a small quantity of balsam of Peru added.

Tincture of cocculus indicus, pure or diluted, may also be applied with good results.

When the parts are markedly eczematous, an ointment of ammoniated mercury or β-naphthol, thirty to sixty grains to the ounce may be used.

Daily shampooing with soap and water, and the twice daily application of a five per cent. carbolic acid lotion, together with the use of a fine-toothed comb, is a safe and efficient method for dispensary practice; as it is, indeed, for any class of patients. [Pg 274]

How are the ova or their shells to be removed from the hair?

By the frequent use of acid or alkaline lotions, such as dilute acetic acid and vinegar, or solutions of sodium carbonate and borax.

Pediculosis Corporis.

Describe the symptoms of pediculosis corporis.

Pediculosis corporis is dependent upon the presence of the pediculus corporis (*pediculus vestimenti*), a larger variety than that infesting the scalp. It is characterized by more or less general itching, together with various inflammatory lesions and excoriations. As the parasites are to be found chiefly in the folds and seams of the clothing, visiting the skin for the purpose of feeding, the various symptoms—the minute hemorrhagic puncta showing the points at which they have been sucking, and the consequent papules, pustules and excoriations—are, therefore, to be found most abundantly on those parts with which the clothing comes closely in contact, as, for instance, around the neck, across the shoulders, around the waist, and down the outside of the thighs. It is uncommon in children.

Fig. 81.

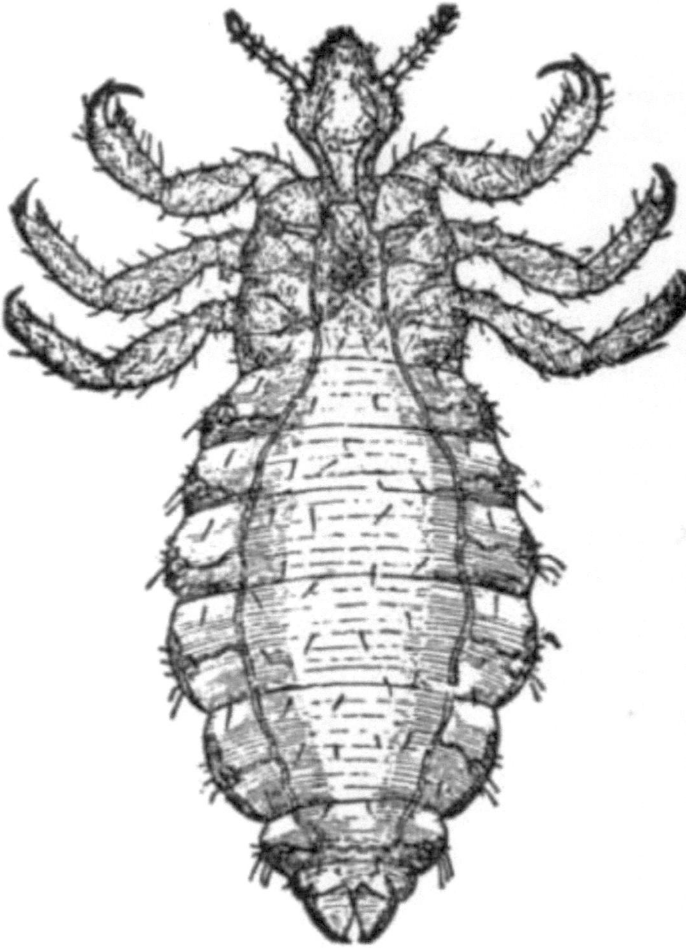

Pediculus Corporis x 25. (*After Duhring.*)

Female. Dorsal surface.

[Pg 275]

State the diagnostic characters of pediculosis corporis.

The presence of the minute hemorrhagic puncta, the multiform character and peculiar distribution of the eruption. Careful search will almost invariably disclose one or more pediculi.

What is the treatment of pediculosis corporis?

The clothing and bed-coverings are to be thoroughly baked or boiled, the pediculi and their ova being in this manner destroyed; a thymol or carbolized boric-acid lotion may be used to relieve the cutaneous irritation.

When attention to the wearing apparel is not immediately practicable, ointments of sulphur and staphisagria, and lotions of carbolic acid, may be advised as temporary measures. The wearing of a bag of loosely woven texture containing some lump sulphur next to the skin is useful in such cases; at the temperature of the body the sulphur undergoes slow oxidation. In hairy individuals the malady is often persistent, due to the fact that ova have become attached to the hair and a new progeny soon hatched out. Continued treatment over a few weeks will usually suffice to rid the patient of their presence.

Pediculosis Pubis.

Describe the symptoms of pediculosis pubis.

Pediculosis pubis is a condition due to the presence of the pediculus pubis, or crab-louse. It is characterized by more or less itching about the genitalia, together with papules, excoriations, and other inflammatory lesions. The amount of irritation varies; it may be slight, or, on the other hand, severe. The parasite, which is the smallest of the three varieties, may be discovered upon close examination seated near the roots of the hairs, clutching the hair, with its head downward and buried in the follicle. The ova may be seen attached to the hair-shafts.

It infests adults chiefly, being in many instances probably contracted through sexual intercourse.

Is the pediculus pubis found upon any other part of the body?

Yes. Although its favorite habitat is the region of the pubes, it [Pg 276] may, in exceptional instances, also infest the axillæ, the sternal region of the male, the beard, eyebrows, and even the eyelashes.

State the diagnostic characters of pediculosis pubis.

The region involved, itching, variable amount of irritation, and, above all, the presence of the pediculi and their ova.

Fig. 82.

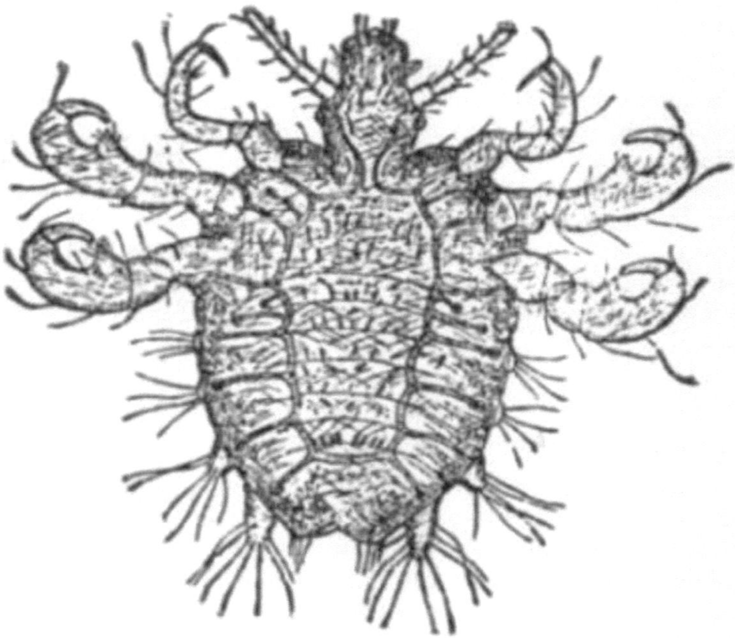

Pediculus Pubis x 25. (*After Duhring.*) Female. Dorsal surface.

Name several applications prescribed for pediculosis pubis.

A lotion of corrosive sublimate, one to four grains to the ounce; infusion of tobacco; a ten to twenty per cent. ointment of oleate of mercury; ammoniated mercury ointment, and a five to ten per cent. β-naphthol ointment. Repeated washings with vinegar or dilute acetic acid, or with alkaline lotions, will free the hairs of the ova.

Cysticercus Cellulosæ.

Describe the cutaneous disturbance produced by the cysticercus cellulosæ.

The presence of cysticerci in the skin and subcutaneous tissue gives rise to pea to hazelnut-sized, rounded, firm, movable tumors which, when developed, may remain unchanged for months. The parasites are disclosed by microscopic examination.

Most of the cases have been observed in Germany. [Pg 277]

Filaria Medinensis.

(*Synonym:* Guinea-worm.)

State the character of the lesions produced by the filaria medinensis.

The young microscopic worm penetrates the skin or deeper tissue, where it grows gradually, finally reaching several inches or more in length and about a half-line in thickness; inflammation is excited and a tumor-like swelling makes its appearance, which, sooner or later, breaks, disclosing the worm. It may also present a cord-like appearance. It is rarely met with outside of tropical countries.

Treatment consists in gradual extraction, or in the injection of a corrosive sublimate solution (1:1000) into the forming tumor. Asafetida internally has been found to be curative, the parasite being destroyed and subsequently absorbed or discharged.

Ixodes.

(*Synonym:* Wood-tick.)

State the character of the cutaneous disturbance produced by the ixodes.

The tick sticks its proboscis into the skin and sucks blood until it is several times its natural size, and then falls off; an urticarial lesion results. If caught in the act the animal should not be forcibly extracted, as its proboscis may be thus broken off and remain in the skin, and give rise to pain and inflammation. It may be made to relinquish its hold by placing on it a drop of an essential oil.

A thymol or carbolized boric-acid lotion will relieve the irritation.

Leptus.

(*Synonym:* Harvest-mite.)

State the characters of the lesion produced by the leptus.

This minute brick-red mite buries itself in the skin, especially about the ankles and feet, giving rise to papules, vesicles and pustules.

Treatment consists of the use of a mild sulphur ointment or of a carbolic-acid lotion. [Pg 278]

Œstrus.

(*Synonym:* Gad, or Bot-fly.)

Describe the cutaneous disturbance produced by the œstrus.

The ova are deposited in the skin, develop and give rise to the formation of furuncle-like tumors with central aperture, through which a sanious discharge exudes; or as the result of the burrowing of the larvæ, irregular serpiginous lines or wheals are produced.

It is chiefly met with in Central and South America.

Larva migrant, or *creeping disease*, is doubtless in this same class. It is characterized by a thread-like linear formation of an erythematous, erythemato-papular, or vesicular nature that gradually extends, the older part disappearing; considerable surface may be covered before the parasite disappears or dies. The treatment consists in endeavoring to destroy the organism by means of excision or caustic applications at the point of its suspected site which is just ahead of the extending line.

Pulex Penetrans.

(*Synonyms:* Sand Flea; Jigger.)

Describe the cutaneous disturbance produced by the pulex penetrans.

This microscopic animal penetrates the skin, especially about the toes, producing an inflammatory swelling, vesicle or pustule, or even ulceration. It is met with in warm and tropical countries.

Treatment consists in extraction. Essential oils are used as a preventive. A carbolic-acid or alkaline lotion relieves irritation.

Cimex Lectularius.

(*Synonym:* Bed-bug.)

Describe the characters of a bed-bug bite.

An inflammatory papule or wheal-like lesion results, somewhat hemorrhagic; the purpuric or hemorrhagic point or spot remains after the swelling subsides, but finally, in the course of several days or a few weeks, disappears.

Treatment consists in the application of alkaline or acid lotions. [Pg 279]

Culex.

(*Synonym:* Gnat; Mosquito.)

Describe the cutaneous disturbance produced by the culex.

It consists of an erythematous spot or a wheal-like lesion.

Alkaline or acid lotions usually give relief.

Pulex Irritans.

(*Synonym:* Common Flea.)

Describe the cutaneous disturbance produced by the pulex irritans.

It consists of an erythematous spot with a minute central hemorrhagic point. In irritable skin, a wheal-like lesion may result.

Treatment consists of applications of camphor or ammonia-water; carbolic acid and thymol lotions are also useful.

[Pg 280]

RELATIVE FREQUENCY OF THE VARIOUS DISEASES OF SKIN AS SHOWN BY THE STATISTICS (123,746 CASES) OF THE

AMERICAN DERMATOLOGICAL ASSOCIATION FOR TEN YEARS, 1878-87.

CLASSIFICATION OF DISEASES.	No. Cases.	% Cases.	CLASSIFICATION OF DISEASES.	No. Cases.	% Cases.
Class I. Disorders of the Glands.			Verruca necrogenica	2	.001
1. OF THE SWEAT GLANDS.			Nævus pigmentosus	88	.064
Hyperidrosis	328	.265	Xerosis	100	.080
Sudamen	268	.216	Ichthyosis	309	.249
Anidrosis	11	.009	Onychauxis	70	.056
Bromidrosis	112	.090	Hypertdichosis	515	.416
Chromidrosis	7	.005	3. OF CONNECTIVE TISSUE.		
Uridrosis	....	....	Sclerema neonatorum	....	....
2. OF THE SEBACEOUS GLANDS	238	.193	Scleroderma	38	0.030
Seborrhœa:	1812	1.47	Morphœa	39	0.031
a. oleosa	367	.296	Elephantiasis	57	0.046
b. sicca	395	.319	Rosacea:	785	0.634
Comedo	1225	.989	a. erythematosa	381	0.308
Cyst	6	.004	b. hypertrophica	58	0.047
a. Milium	225	.183	Frambœsia	22	0.018
b. Steatoma	151	.122	**Class V. Atrophies.**		
Asteatosis	8	.006	1. OF PIGMENT.		

Class II. Inflammations.			Leucoderma	77	0.062
Exanthemata	1770	1.43	Albinismus	9	0.008
Erythema simplex	1064	.859	Vitiligo	191	0.155
Erythema multiforme:	915	.730	Canities	43	0.035
a. papulosum	325	.262	2. OF HAIR.		
b. bullosum	37	.029	Alopecia	926	0.749
c. nodosum	82	.066	Alopecia furfuracea	830	0.67
Urticaria	2994	2.47	Alopecia areata	794	0.641
pigmentosa	1	.0008	Atrophia pilorum propria	23	0.019
[E]Dermatitis:	1720	1.39	Trichorexis nodosa	3	0.002
a. traumatica	468	.378	3. OF NAIL	26	0.021
b. venenata	616	.498	Atrophia unguis	19	0.015
c. calorica	224	.187	4. OF CUTIS	6	0.005
d. medicamentosa	108	.087	Atrophia senilis	15	0.013
e. gangrænosa	8	.006	Atrophia maculosa et striata	23	0.019
Erysipelas	1026	.829	**Class VI. New Growths.**		
Furunculus	2129	1.72	1. OF CONNECTIVE TISSUE.	1	0.0008
Anthrax	252	.203	Keloid	152	0.124
Phlegmona diffusa	265	.215	Cicatrix	89	0.065

Pustula maligna	197	.159	Fibroma	93	0.075
Herpes simplex	2057	1.66	Neuroma	11	0.009
Herpes zoster	1428	1.15	Xanthoma	69	0.056
Dermatitis herpetiformis	41	.033	2. OF MUSCULAR TISSUE.		
Psoriasis	4131	3.34	Myoma	1	0.0008
Pityriasis maculuta et circinata	71	.057	3. OF VESSELS.		
Dermatitis exfoliativa	16	.012	Angioma	462	0.373
Pityriasis rubra	44	.032	Angioma pigmentosum et atrophicum	13	0.010
Lichen:	144	.116	Angioma cavernosum	22	0.018
a. planus	154	.124	Lymphangioma	16	.012
b. ruber	27	.021	4. Mycosis fongoide	1	.0008
Eczema:	37661	30.43	Rhinoscleroma	3	.002
a. erythematosum	....	....	Lupus erythematosus	477	.385
b. papulosum	....	....	Lupus vulgaris	536	.433
c. vesiculosum	....	....	Scrofuloderma	663	.536
d. madidans	....	....	Syphiloderma:	13888	11.22
e. pustulosum	....	....	a. erythematosum	....	....
f. rubrum	....	....	b. papulosum	....	....
g. squamosum	....	....	c. pustulosum	....	....
Prurigo	34	.027	d. tuberculosum	....	....

Acne	9077	7.34	e. gummatosum	....	....
Acne rosacea	398	.321	Lepra:	24	.020
Sycosis	227	.185	a. tuberosa	7	.005
Impetigo	1769	1.43	b. maculosa	4	.003
Impetigo contagiosa	600	.485	c. anæsthetica	6	.004
Impetigo herpetiformis	10	.009	Carcinoma	1068	.863
Ecthyma	726	.587	Sarcoma	55	.044
Pemphigus	183	.148	**Class VII. Neuroses.**		
Ulcers	3021	2.44	Hyperæsthesia:	4	.003
Class III. Hemorrhages.			a. Pruritus	2716	2.12
Purpura:	341	.275	b. Dermatalgia	11	.009
a. simplex	181	.145	Anæsthesia	22	.018
b. hæmorrhagica	49	.039	**Class VIII. Parasitic Affections.**		
Class IV. Hypertrophies.			1. VEGETABLE.		
1. OF PIGMENT.			Tinea favosa	354	.286
Lentigo	127	.103	Tinea trichophytina:	2289	1.85
Chloasma	560	.452	a. circinata	705	.569
2. OF EPIDERMAL AND PAPILLARY LAYERS.			b. tonsurans	675	.545
Keratosis:	94	.076	c. sycosis	365	.295

a. pilaris	103	.083	Tinea versicolor	1263	1.02
b. senilis	68	.055	2. ANIMAL.		
Molluscum epitheliale	172	.139	Scabies	3192	2.58
Callositas	110	.090	Pediculosis capillitii	2579	2.09
Clavus	84	.068	Pediculosis corporis	1704	1.38
Cornu cutaneum	42	.034	Pediculosis pubis	436	.352
Verruca	1252	1.09	Total	123746	

[E] Indicating affections of this class not properly included under other titles.

INDEX.

SAUNDERS' TEXT-BOOKS CONTINUE TO GAIN

The list of text-books recommended in the various colleges again shows a **decided gain for the Saunders publications**. During the present college year, in the list of recommended books published by 164 colleges (the other 23 have not published lists), the Saunders books are mentioned 3278 times, as against 3054 the previous year—**an increase of 224**. In other words, in each of the medical colleges in this country an average of 20 (18-2/5 the previous year) of the teaching books employed are publications issued by W. B. Saunders Company. That this increase is not due alone to the publication of new text-books, but rather to a most gratifying increase in the recommendation of text-books recognized as standards, is at once evident from the following: Ashton's Gynecology shows an increase of 19; DaCosta's Surgery, an increase of 12; Hirst's Obstetrics, 14; Howell's Physiology, 25; Jackson on the Eye, 16; Sahli's Diagnostic Methods, 11; Scudder's Fractures, 11; Stengel's Pathology, 13; Stelwagon on the Skin, 11. These are but examples of similar remarkable gains throughout the entire list, and is undoubted evidence that the **Saunders text-books are recognized as the best**.

A Complete Catalogue of our Publications will be Sent upon Request

Bandler's

Medical Gynecology

Medical Gynecology. By S. Wyllis Bandler, M.D., Adjunct. Professor of Diseases of Women, New York Post-Graduate Medical School and Hospital. Octavo of 680 pages, with 135 original illustrations. Cloth, $5.00 net; Half Morocco, $6.50 net.

JUST READY – EXCLUSIVELY MEDICAL GYNECOLOGY

This new work by Dr. Bandler is just the book that the physician engaged in general practice has long needed. It is truly *the practitioner's gynecology* – planned for him, written for him, and illustrated for him. There are many gynecologic conditions that do not call for operative treatment; yet, because of lack of that special knowledge required for their diagnosis and treatment, the general practitioner has been unable to treat them intelligently. This work gives just the information the practitioner needs. It not only deals with those conditions amenable to non-operative treatment, but it also tells how to recognize those diseases demanding operative treatment, so that the practitioner will be enabled to advise his patient at a time when operation will be attended with the most favorable results. The chapter on Pessaries is especially full and excellent, the proper manner of introducing the pessary being clearly described and illustrated with original pictures that show plainly the correct technic of this procedure. The chapters on Vaginal and Abdominal Massage, and particularly that on Artificial Hyperemia and Anemia, are extremely valuable to the practitioner. They express the very latest advances in these methods of treatment. Hydrotherapy, especially the Ferguson and Nauheim baths, are treated *in extenso*, and Electrotherapy receives the full consideration its importance merits. Pain as a symptom and its alleviation is dealt with in an unusually practical way, its value as an aid in diagnosis being emphasized. Gonorrhea and Syphilis and their many complications are treated in detail, every care being taken to have these sections – of special interest to the practitioner – complete in every particular. Other chapters of great importance are those on Constipation, Sterility, Associated Nervous Conditions in Gynecology, and Pregnancy and Abortion.

Kelly and Noble's Gynecology

and Abdominal Surgery

Gynecology and Abdominal Surgery. Edited by Howard A. Kelly, M.D., Professor of Gynecology in Johns Hopkins University; and Charles P. Noble, M.D., Clinical Professor of Gynecology in the Woman's Medical College, Philadelphia. Two imperial octavo volumes of 900 pages each, containing 650 illustrations, mostly original. Per volume: Cloth, $8.00 net; Half Morocco, $9.50 net.

BOTH VOLUMES NOW READY

WITH 650 ORIGINAL ILLUSTRATIONS BY HERMANN BECKER

AND MAX BRÖDEL

In view of the intimate association of gynecology with abdominal surgery the editors have combined these two important subjects in one work. For this reason the work will be doubly valuable, for not only the gynecologist and general practitioner will find it an exhaustive treatise, but the surgeon also will find here the latest technic of the various abdominal operations. It possesses a number of valuable features not to be found in any other publication covering the same fields. It contains a chapter upon the bacteriology and one upon the pathology of gynecology, dealing fully with the scientific basis of gynecology. In no other work can this information, prepared by specialists, be found as separate chapters. There is a large chapter devoted entirely to *medical gynecology*, written especially for the physician engaged in general practice. Heretofore the general practitioner was compelled to search through an entire work in order to obtain the information desired. *Abdominal surgery* proper, as distinct from gynecology, is fully treated, embracing operations upon the stomach, upon the intestines, upon the liver and bile-ducts, upon the pancreas and spleen, upon the kidney, ureter, bladder, and the peritoneum. Special attention has been given to *modern technic* and illustrations of the very highest order have been used to make clear the various steps of the operations. Indeed, the illustrations are truly magnificent, being the work of *Mr. Hermann Becker* and *Mr. Max Brödel*, of the Johns Hopkins Hospital.

Ashton's

Practice of Gynecology

The Practice of Gynecology. By W. Easterly Ashton, M.D., LL.D., Professor of Gynecology in the Medico-Chirurgical College, Philadelphia. Handsome octavo volume of 1096 pages, containing 1057 original line drawings. Cloth, $6.50 net; Half Morocco, $8.00 net.

RECENTLY ISSUED – NEW (3d) EDITION

THREE EDITIONS IN EIGHTEEN MONTHS

Three editions of this work have been demanded in eighteen months. Among the new additions are: Colonic lavage and flushing, Hirst's treatment for vaginismus, Dudley's treatment of cystocele, Montgomery's round ligament operation, Chorio-epithelioma of the Uterus, Passive Incontinence of the Urine, and Moynihan's methods in Intestinal Anastomosis. Nothing is left to be taken for granted, the author not only telling his readers in every instance what should be done, but also precisely *how to do it*. A distinctly original feature of the book is the illustrations, numbering about one thousand line drawings made especially under the author's personal supervision from actual apparatus, living models, and dissections on the cadaver. These line drawings show in detail the procedures and operations without obscuring their purpose by unnecessary and unimportant anatomic surroundings.

Howard A. Kelly, M.D.

Professor of Gynecology, Johns Hopkins University.

"It is different from anything that has as yet appeared. The illustrations are particularly clear and satisfactory. One specially good feature is the pains with which you describe so many *details* so often left to the imagination."

Charles B. Penrose, M.D.,

Formerly Professor of Gynecology, University of Pennsylvania.

"I know of no book that goes so thoroughly and satisfactorily into all the *details* of everything connected with the subject. In this respect your book differs from the others."

George M. Edebohls, M.D.

Professor of Diseases of Women, New York Post-Graduate Medical School. "I have looked it through and must congratulate you upon having produced a text-book most admirably adapted to *teach* gynecology to those who must get their knowledge, even to the minutest and most elementary details, from books."

Webster's

Diseases *of* Women

Diseases of Women. By J. Clarence Webster, M.D. (Edin.), F.R.C.P.E., Professor of Gynecology and Obstetrics in Rush Medical College. Octavo of 712 pages, with 372 illustrations. Cloth, $7.00 net; Half Morocco, $8.50 net.

RECENTLY ISSUED—FOR THE PRACTITIONER

Dr. Webster has written this work *especially for the general practitioner*, discussing the clinical features of the subject in their widest relations to general practice rather than from the standpoint of specialism. The magnificent illustrations, three hundred and seventy-two in number, are nearly all original. Drawn by expert anatomic artists under Dr. Webster's direct supervision, they portray the anatomy of the parts and the steps in the operations with rare clearness and exactness.

Howard A. Kelly, M.D., *Professor of Gynecology, Johns Hopkins University.*

"It is undoubtedly one of the best works which has been put on the market within recent years, showing from start to finish Dr. Webster's well-known thoroughness. The illustrations are also of the highest order."

Webster's Obstetrics

A Text-Book of Obstetrics. By J. Clarence Webster, M.D. (Edin.), Professor of Obstetrics and Gynecology in Rush Medical College. Octavo of 767 pages, illustrated. Cloth, $5.00 net; Half Morocco, $6.50 net.

RECENTLY ISSUED

Medical Record, New York

"The author's remarks on asepsis and antisepsis are admirable, the chapter on eclampsia is full of good material, and ... the book can be cordially recommended as a safe guide."

Cullen's

Uterine Adenomyoma

Uterine Adenomyoma. By Thomas S. Cullen, M.D., Associate Professor of Gynecology, Johns Hopkins University. Octavo of 275 pages, with original illustrations by Hermann Becker and August Horn. Cloth, $5.00 net.

JUST READY

Dr. Cullen's large clinical experience and his extensive original work along the lines of gynecologic pathology have enabled him to present his subject with originality and precision. The work gives the early literature on adenomyoma, traces the disease through its various stages, and then gives the detailed findings in a large number of cases personally examined by the author. Formerly the physician and surgeon were unable to determine the cause of uterine bleeding, but after following closely the clinical course of the disease, Dr. Cullen has found that the majority of these cases can be diagnosed clinically. The results of these observations he presents in this work. The entire subject of adenomyoma is dealt with from the standpoint of the pathologist, the clinician, and the surgeon. The superb illustrations are the work of Mr. Hermann Becker and Mr. August Horn, of the Johns Hopkins Hospital.

The American

Text-Book *of* Obstetrics

Recently Issued—New (2d) Edition

The American Text-Book of Obstetrics. In two volumes. Edited by Richard C. Norris, M.D.; Art Editor, Robert L. Dickinson, M.D. Two octavos of about 600 pages each; nearly 900 illustrations, including 49 colored and half-tone plates. Per volume: Cloth, $3.50 net; Half Morocco, $4.50 net.

American Journal of the Medical Sciences

"As an authority, as a book of reference, as a 'working book' for the student or practitioner, we commend it because we believe there is no better."

Hirst's

Diseases of Women

A Text-Book of Diseases of Women. By Barton Cooke Hirst, M.D., Professor of Obstetrics, University of Pennsylvania; Gynecologist to the Howard, the Orthopedic, and the Philadelphia Hospitals. Octavo of 745 pages, 701 illustrations, many in colors. Cloth, $5.00 net; Half Morocco, $6.50 net.

RECENTLY ISSUED—NEW (2d) EDITION

WITH 701 ORIGINAL ILLUSTRATIONS

The new edition of this work has just been issued after a careful revision. As diagnosis and treatment are of the greatest importance in considering diseases of women, particular attention has been devoted to these divisions. To this end, also, the work has been magnificently illuminated with 701 illustrations, for the most part original photographs and water-colors of actual clinical cases accumulated during the past fifteen years. The palliative treatment, as well as the radical operative, is fully described, enabling the general practitioner to treat many of his own patients without referring them to a specialist. The author's extensive experience renders this work of unusual value.

OPINIONS OF THE MEDICAL PRESS

Medical Record, New York

"Its merits can be appreciated only by a careful perusal.... Nearly one hundred pages are devoted to technic, this chapter being in some respects superior to the descriptions in many text-books."

Boston Medical and Surgical Journal

"The author has given special attention to diagnosis and treatment throughout the book, and has produced a practical treatise which should be of the greatest value to the student, the general practitioner, and the specialist."

Medical News, New York

"Office treatment is given a due amount of consideration, so that the work will be as useful to the non-operator as to the specialist."

Hirst's

Text-Book of Obstetrics

New (5th) Edition, Revised

A Text-Book of Obstetrics. By Barton Cooke Hirst, M.D., Professor of Obstetrics in the University of Pennsylvania. Handsome octavo, 899 pages, with 746 illustrations, 39 in colors. Cloth, $5.00 net; Sheep or Half Morocco, $6.50 net.

RECENTLY ISSUED

Immediately on its publication this work took its place as the leading text-book on the subject. Both in this country and abroad it is recognized as the most satisfactorily written and clearly illustrated work on obstetrics in the language. The illustrations form one of the features of the book. They are numerous and the most of them are original. In this edition the book has been thoroughly revised. More attention has been given to the diseases of the genital organs associated with or following childbirth. Many of the old illustrations have been replaced by better ones, and there have been added a number entirely new. The work treats the subject from a clinical standpoint.

OPINIONS OF THE MEDICAL PRESS

British Medical Journal

"The popularity of American text-books in this country is one of the features of recent years. The popularity is probably chiefly due to the great superiority of their illustration over those of the English text-books. The illustrations in Dr. Hirst's volume are far more numerous and far better executed, and therefore more instructive, than those commonly found in the works of writers on obstetrics in our own country."

Bulletin of Johns Hopkins Hospital

"The work is an admirable one in every sense of the word, concisely but comprehensively written."

The Medical Record, New York

"The illustrations are numerous and are works of art, many of them appearing for the first time. The author's style, though condensed, is singularly clear, so that it is never necessary to re-read a sentence in order to grasp the meaning. As a true model of what a modern text-book on obstetrics should be, we feel justified in affirming that Dr. Hirst's book is without a rival."

Penrose's

Diseases of Women

Sixth Revised Edition

A Text-Book of Diseases of Women. By Charles B. Penrose, M.D., Ph.D., formerly Professor of Gynecology in the University of Pennsylvania; Surgeon to the Gynecean Hospital, Philadelphia. Octavo volume of 550 pages, with 225 fine original illustrations. Cloth $3.75 net.

JUST ISSUED

Regularly every year a new edition of this excellent text-book is called for, and it appears to be in as great favor with physicians as with students. Indeed, this book has taken its place as the ideal work for the general practitioner. The author presents the best teaching of modern gynecology, untrammeled by antiquated ideas and methods. In every case the most modern and progressive technique is adopted, and the main points are made clear by excellent illustrations. The new edition has been carefully revised, much new matter has been added, and a number of new original illustrations have been introduced. In its revised form this volume continues to be an admirable exposition of the present status of gynecologic practice.

PERSONAL AND PRESS OPINIONS

Howard A. Kelly, M.D.,

Professor of Gynecology and Obstetrics, Johns Hopkins University, Baltimore.

"I shall value very highly the copy of Penrose's 'Diseases of Women' received. I have already recommended it to my class as the best book."

L.E. Montgomery, M.D.,

Professor of Gynecology, Jefferson Medical College, Philadelphia.

"The copy of 'A Text-Book of Diseases of Women' by Penrose received to-day. I have looked over it and admire it very much. I have no doubt it will have a large sale, as it justly merits."

Bristol Medico-Chirurgical Journal

"This is an excellent work which goes straight to the mark.... The book may be taken as a trustworthy exposition of modern gynecology."

Gives a Maximum Amount of Matter in a Minimum Space, and at the Lowest Possible Cost

WITH 2000 NEW TERMS

The immediate success of this work is due to the special features that distinguish it from other books of its kind. It gives a maximum of matter in a minimum space and at the lowest possible cost. Though it is practically unabridged, yet by the use of thin bible paper and flexible morocco binding it is only 1-1/4 inches thick. In this new edition the book has been thoroughly revised, and upward of two thousand new terms have been added, thus bringing the book absolutely up to date. The book contains hundreds of terms not to be found in any other dictionary, over 100 original tables, and many handsome illustrations.

PERSONAL OPINIONS

Howard A. Kelly, M.D.,

Professor of Gynecology, Johns Hopkins University, Baltimore.

"Dr. Borland's dictionary is admirable. It is so well gotten up and of such convenient size. No errors have been found in my use of it."

J. Collins Warren, M.D., LL.D., F.R.C.S. (Hon.)

Professor of Surgery, Harvard Medical School.

"I regard it as a valuable aid to my medical literary work. It is very complete and of convenient size to handle comfortably. I use it in preference to any other."

Garrigues'

Diseases of Women

Third Edition, Thoroughly Revised

A Text-Book of Diseases of Women. By Henry J. Garrigues, A.M., M.D., Gynecologist to St. Mark's Hospital and to the German Dispensary, New York City. Handsome octavo, 756 pages, with 367 engravings and colored plates. Cloth, $4.50 net; Sheep or Half Morocco, $6.00 net.

The first two editions of this work met with a most appreciative reception by the medical profession both in this country and abroad. In this edition the entire work has been carefully and thoroughly revised, and considerable new matter added, bringing the work precisely down to date. Many new illustrations have been introduced, thus greatly increasing the value of the book both as a text-book and book of reference.

Thad. A. Reamy, M.D., *Professor of Gynecology, Medical College of Ohio.*

"One of the best text-books for students and practitioners which has been published in the English language; it is condensed, clear, and comprehensive. The profound learning and great clinical experience of the distinguished author find expression in this book."

American

Text-Book of Gynecology

American Text-Book of Gynecology. Medical and Surgical. Edited by J. M. Baldy, M.D., Professor of Gynecology, Philadelphia Polyclinic. Imperial octavo of 718 pages, with 341 text-illustrations and 38 plates. Cloth, $6.00 net; Half Morocco, $7.50 net.

SECOND REVISED EDITION

This volume is thoroughly practical in its teachings, and is intended to be a working text-book for physicians and students. Many of the most important subject are considered from an entirely new standpoint, and are grouped together in a manner somewhat foreign to the accepted custom.

Boston Medical and Surgical Journal

"The most complete exponent of gynecology that we have. No subject seems to have been neglected."

Dorland's

Modern Obstetrics

Modern Obstetrics: General and Operative. By W. A. Newman Dorland, A.M., M.D., Assistant Instructor in Obstetrics, University of Pennsylvania; Associate in Gynecology in the Philadelphia Polyclinic. Handsome octavo volume of 797 pages, with 201 illustrations. Cloth, $4.00 net.

Second Edition, Revised and Greatly Enlarged

In this edition the book has been entirely rewritten and very greatly enlarged. Among the new subjects introduced are the surgical treatment of puerperal sepsis, infant mortality, placental transmission of diseases, serum-therapy of puerperal sepsis, etc.

Journal of the American Medical Association

"This work deserves commendation, and that it has received what it deserves at the hands of the profession is attested by the fact that a second edition is called for within such a short time. Especially deserving of praise is the chapter on puerperal sepsis."

Davis' Obstetric and

Gynecologic Nursing

Obstetric and Gynecologic Nursing. By Edward P. Davis, A.M., M.D., Professor of Obstetrics in the Jefferson Medical College and Philadelphia Polyclinic; Obstetrician and Gynecologist, Philadelphia Hospital. 12mo of 436 pages, illustrated. Buckram, $1.75 net.

JUST ISSUED—THIRD REVISED EDITION

This volume gives a very clear and accurate idea of the manner to meet the conditions arising during obstetric and gynecologic nursing. The third edition has been thoroughly revised.

The Lancet, London

"Not only nurses, but even newly qualified medical men, would learn a great deal by a perusal of this book. It is written in a clear and pleasant style, and is a work we can recommend."

Schäffer *and* Edgar's

Labor and Operative Obstetrics

Atlas and Epitome of Labor and Operative Obstetrics. By Dr. O. Schäffer, of Heidelberg. *From the Fifth Revised and Enlarged German Edition.* Edited, with additions, by J. Clifton Edgar, M.D., Professor of Obstetrics and Clinical Midwifery, Cornell University Medical School, New York. With 14 lithographic plates in colors, 139 other illustrations, and 111 pages of text. Cloth, $2.00 net. *In Saunders' Hand-Atlas Series.*

This book presents the act of parturition and the various obstetric operations in a series of easily understood illustrations, accompanied by a text treating the subject from a practical standpoint.

American Medicine

"The method of presenting obstetric operations is admirable. The drawings, representing original work, have the commendable merit of illustrating instead of confusing."

Schäffer *and* Edgar's

Obstetric Diagnosis and Treatment

Atlas and Epitome of Obstetric Diagnosis and Treatment. By Dr. O. Schäffer, of Heidelberg. *From the Second Revised German Edition.*Edited, with additions, by J. Clifton Edgar, M.D., Professor of Obstetrics and Clinical Midwifery, Cornell University Medical

School, N.Y. With 122 colored figures on 56 plates, 38 text-cuts, and 315 pages of text. Cloth, $3.00 net. *In Saunders' Hand-Atlas Series.*

This book treats particularly of obstetric operations, and, besides the wealth of beautiful lithographic illustrations, contains an extensive text of great value. This text deals with the practical, clinical side of the subject.

New York Medical Journal

"The illustrations are admirably executed, as they are in all of these atlases, and the text can safely be commended, not only as elucidatory of the plates, but as expounding the scientific midwifery of to-day."

Schäffer and Norris'

Gynecology

Atlas and Epitome of Gynecology. By Dr. O. Schäffer, of Heidelberg. *From the Second Revised and Enlarged German Edition.* Edited, with additions, by Richard C. Norris, A.M., M.D., Assistant Professor of Obstetrics in the University of Pennsylvania. 207 colored figures on 90 plates, 65 text-cuts, and 308 pages of text. Cloth, $3.50 net. *In Saunders' Hand-Atlas Series.*

American Journal of the Medical Sciences

"Of the illustrations it is difficult to speak in too high terms of approval. They are so clear and true to nature that the accompanying explanations are almost superfluous. We commend it most earnestly."

Galbraith's

Four Epochs of Woman's Life

Second Revised Edition—Recently Issued

The Four Epochs of Woman's Life: A Study in Hygiene. By Anna M. Galbraith, M.D., Fellow of the New York Academy of Medicine, etc. With an Introductory Note by John M. Musser, M.D. Professor of Clinical Medicine, University of Pennsylvania. 12 mo of 247 pages. Cloth $1.50 net.

MAIDENHOOD, MARRIAGE, MATERNITY, MENOPAUSE

In this instructive work are stated, in a modest, pleasing, and conclusive manner, those truths of which every woman should have a thorough knowledge. Written, as it is, for the laity, the subject is discussed in language readily grasped even by those most unfamiliar with medical subjects.

Birmingham Medical Review, England

"We do not as a rule care for medical books written for the instruction of the public. But we must admit that the advice in Dr. Galbraith's work is in the main wise and wholesome."

Schäffer and Webster's

Operative Gynecology

Atlas and Epitome of Operative Gynecology. By Dr. O. Schäffer, of Heidelberg. Edited, with additions, by J. Clarence Webster, M.D. (Edin.), F.R.C.P.E., Professor of Obstetrics and Gynecology in Rush Medical College, in affiliation with the University of Chicago. 42 colored lithographic plates, many text-cuts, a number in colors, and 138 pages of text. *In Saunders' Hand-Atlas Series.* Cloth, $3.00 net.

RECENTLY ISSUED

Much patient endeavor has been expended by the author, the artist, and the lithographer in the preparation of the plates for this Atlas. They are based on hundreds of photographs taken from nature, and illustrate most faithfully the various surgical situations. Dr. Schäffer has made a specialty of demonstrating by illustrations.

Medical Record, New York

"The volume should prove most helpful to students and others in grasping details usually to be acquired only in the amphitheater itself."

DeLee's Obstetrics for Nurses

Obstetrics for Nurses. By Joseph B. DeLee, M.D., Professor of Obstetrics in the Northwestern University Medical School, Chicago; Lecturer in the Nurses' Training Schools of Mercy, Wesley, Provident, Cook County, and Chicago Lying-in Hospitals. 12mo of 512 pages, fully illustrated.

Cloth, $2.50 net.

JUST ISSUED—NEW (3d) EDITION

While Dr. DeLee has written his work especially for nurses, the practitioner will also find it useful and instructive, since the duties of a nurse often devolve upon him in the early years of his practice. The illustrations are nearly all original and represent photographs taken from actual scenes. The text is the result of the author's many years' experience in lecturing to the nurses of five different training schools.

J. Clifton Edgar, M.D.,

Professor of Obstetrics and Clinical Midwifery, Cornell University, New York.

"It is far and away the best that has come to my notice, and I shall take great pleasure in recommending it to my nurses, and students as well."

American Pocket Dictionary **Recently issued—5th Ed.**

The American Pocket Medical Dictionary. Edited by W. A. Newman Dorland, A.M., M.D., Assistant Obstetrician to the Hospital of the University of Pennsylvania; Fellow of the American Academy of Medicine. With 578 pages. Full leather, limp, with gold edges, $1.00 net; with patent thumb index, $1.25 net.

James W. Holland. M.D.,

Professor of Chemistry and Toxicology, at the Jefferson Medical College, Philadelphia.

"I am struck at once with admiration at the compact size and attractive exterior. I can recommend it to our students without reserve."

Cragin's Gynecology **Recently Issued—New (6th) Ed.**

Essentials of Gynecology. By Edwin B. Cragin, M.D., Professor of Obstetrics, College of Physicians and Surgeons, New York. Crown octavo, 240 pages, 62 illustrations. Cloth, $1.00 net. *In Saunders' Question-Compend Series.*

The Medical Record, New York

"A handy volume and a distinct improvement on students' compends in general. No author who was not himself a practical gynecologist could have consulted the student's needs so thoroughly as Dr. Cragin has done."

Boisliniere's Obstetric Accidents, Emergencies, and Operations

Obstetric Accidents, Emergencies, and Operations. By the late L. Ch. Boisliniere, M.D., Emeritus Professor of Obstetrics, St. Louis Medical College; Consulting Physician, St. Louis Female Hospital. 381 pages, illustrated. Cloth, $2.00 net.

British Medical Journal

"It is clearly and concisely written, and is evidently the work of a teacher and practitioner of large experience. Its merit lies in the judgment which comes from experience."

Ashton's Obstetrics **Recently Issued—New (6th) Ed.**

Essentials of Obstetrics. By W. Easterly Ashton, M.D., Professor of Gynecology in the Medico-Chirurgical College, Philadelphia. Crown octavo, 252 pages, 75 illustrations. Cloth, $1.00 net. *In Saunders' Question-Compend Series.*

Southern Practitioner

"An excellent little volume, containing correct and practical knowledge. An admirable compend, and the best condensation we have seen."

Barton and Wells' Medical Thesaurus

A Thesaurus of Medical Words and Phrases. By Wilfred M. Barton, M.D., Assistant to Professor of Materia Medica and Therapeutics, Georgetown University, Washington, D.C.; and Walter A. Wells, M.D., Demonstrator of Laryngology, Georgetown University, Washington, D.C. 12mo of 534 pages. Flexible leather, $2.50 net; with thumb index, $3.00 net.